A Mighty Foe

There are 100,000,000,000,000 cells in the human body ... but the amazing immune system is capable of:

- Recognizing a foreign invader

- Mobilizing an attack to destroy the invader

- Producing millions of different antibodies—each one designed to attack a specific invader

- Recognizing and attacking tumor cells

- Remembering diseases the body has previously been exposed to and keeping antibodies circulating to prevent a second attack.

... and operating on 24-hour alert to keep you healthy!

Other Avon Books by
Eve Potts and Marion Morra

CHOICES: REALISTIC ALTERNATIVES IN
CANCER TREATMENT

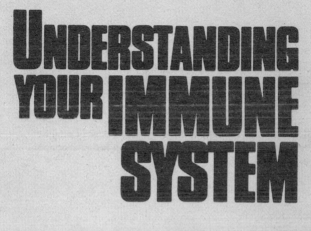

UNDERSTANDING YOUR IMMUNE SYSTEM

EVE POTTS AND MARION MORRA

AVON
PUBLISHERS OF BARD, CAMELOT, DISCUS AND FLARE BOOKS

This book was current to the best of the authors' knowledge at publication, but before acting on information herein, the consumer should verify information with the appropriate physician or agency.

UNDERSTANDING YOUR IMMUNE SYSTEM is an original publication of Avon Books. This work has never before appeared in book form.

AVON BOOKS
A division of
The Hearst Corporation
1790 Broadway
New York, New York 10019

First Avon Printing, June 1986

Printed in the U. S. A.

K-R 10 9 8 7 6 5 4 3 2 1

This book is dedicated to all the scientists, researchers, and doctors who are working in the vast, complicated, and, in many cases, uncharted, areas of immunological research. It is their hard work, insights, and reporting that have served as our sources of information as gleaned from the latest research findings presented in medical journals and at medical conferences, as well as from personal discussion. This book could not have been developed without their generous help. We are especially grateful for the help of Dr. Marc Ernstoff of the Yale School of Medicine. We are also indebted to Deborah Jurkowitz of Avon and to our editor, Ellen LaBarbera, for their guidance and assistance.

Our most special thanks are reserved for Robert Potts for his long-standing patience, understanding, and loyalty and to the rest of our families for their continuing help and support.

Contents

Illustrations and Tables

Foreword

When we stand and gaze at the stars, we marvel at the vastness and complexity of our solar system, little appreciating that our inner space—the space within our own bodies—is even more complex and mysterious. New clues about the immune system are being gathered at a rapid pace in research and biology labs across the world. New discoveries are being added daily to our knowledge about this most intricate of all human systems. There is no doubt that more information about experiments dealing with various aspects of immunity have been published in the last 3 years than in the previous 50 years.

Yet a full understanding of the biomedical technology, the true mechanics of the immune system, and the intricacies of the substances and forces that create immunity are still in the process of being discovered. If there is one thing on which the entire scientific community can agree, it is that the immune system is far from being fully understood. However, much of the information about the immune system is generally accepted by scientists and doctors. Far from being the result of a conspiracy of silence, the subject simply has not been fully explored for the layman. As medical writers we realized that the basic information, as well as results of the current research that is available in the medical literature, needed to be made available to the general public.

We hope that the facts and information in this book will help you to a better understanding of your immune system—how remarkable it is and how you can make it even stronger. However, since this book is designed as a health-education service, it is not intended as a substitute for medical advice from your physician or other health professionals.

Testing Your Immunity Knowledge

TRUE	FALSE		THE REAL ANSWER
____	____	Nursing gives a baby immunity.	True. Colostrum, passed on in early nursing feedings, gives protection for about 6 months. (See p. 57.)
____	____	Our emotions and our brains have an effect on our immune systems.	True. Scientists have found that many illnesses have a mind-body link. (See p. 58.)
____	____	A person may be able to control his or her own immune system.	True. Tests in animals show that it may be possible to control the immune system through conditioned response. (See p. 60.)
____	____	Hypnosis and acupuncture can produce anesthesia.	False. However, both can produce an absence of the ability to feel pain. (See p. 69.)
____	____	Pain can suppress normal functioning of the immune system.	True. Pain, particularly after surgery, can suppress the immune system and delay recovery. (See p. 49.)
____	____	The appendix is part of the immune system.	True. Though its specific role is unknown, the concentration of lymphoid tissue indicates it plays a role in the immune system. (See p. 7.)
____	____	During a full moon, people have higher metabolism rates.	True. Researchers have also found that patients with bleeding ulcers, epilepsy, and angina are more likely to suffer a crisis during a full moon than at other times of the month. (See p. 41.)
____	____	Dinosaurs had arthritis.	True. Skeletons of dinosaurs, dating back 200 million years, show evidence of osteoarthritis. (See p. 200.)

True	False		The Real Answer
____	____	Rheumatoid arthritis is caused by an overactive immune system.	True. Investigators believe that it is due to an overproduction of antibody, which results in chronic inflammation. (See p. 199.)
____	____	Too much zinc in the diet weakens immunity.	False. A zinc *shortage* in the diet can weaken body immunity. (See p. 54.)
____	____	You never really recover from herpes.	True. The virus "hides" in the body, and infection can recur many years later. The virus is infectious until the sores are completely healed. (See p. 155.)
____	____	The body makes a different antibody for each disease.	True. The immune system is capable of turning out millions of kinds of antibodies—each one specifically designed against one substance. (See p. 16.)
____	____	The red rash of measles is the immune system at work.	True. The virus at this point is all but dead. The rash is the result of the immune system combating the virus. (See p. 164.)
____	____	Wet chilling and wet feet bring on colds.	False. Researchers find little or no connection between wet chilling and catching cold. (See p. 147.)
____	____	Someday soon, we'll have a vaccine against colds.	False. Many scientists feel that with more than 200 infectious agents involved, it would be almost impossible to produce one general cold vaccine. (See p. 148.)
____	____	Animals never get flu.	False. The first flu virus was isolated from a pig in 1930. Many of the flu viruses appear to originate with birds, especially ducks. (See p. 149.)

TRUE	FALSE		THE REAL ANSWER
——	——	Viruses are so small that about 10,000 could fit on the period at the end of this sentence.	True. Viruses are about 1/100th the size of bacteria. (See p. 137.)
——	——	Selenium can slow down the growth of tumors.	False. However, studies with mice indicate that selenium given before the onset of cancer can prevent tumors from developing. (See p. 97.)
——	——	Right-handed people are more susceptible to autoimmune diseases.	False. Left-handers seem to be more sensitive to autoimmune diseases. (See p. 60.)
——	——	Allergies are not related to the immune system.	False. The wheezing, sneezing, runny nose, itchy eyes, rashes, and bumps are the result of the immune system responding to a false alarm or an overreaction to a true alarm. (See p. 194.)
——	——	Plants manufacture poisonous substances.	True. They create them apparently to defend themselves against the millions of insects, bacteria, and fungi. It is estimated that we are exposed to 10,000 times the amount of natural pesticides as of man-made pesticides. (See p. 39.)
——	——	Licorice may be a factor in the high cancer rate among smokers.	True. Licorice depletes potassium levels. Thus, since it is a widely used additive in tobacco products, it may be a contributing factor in the high cancer rate among smokers. (See p. 96.)
——	——	The older you are, the less effective your immune system is.	True. The capacity of the immune system to respond is lower in older animals and older people. (See p. 23.)

TRUE	FALSE		THE REAL ANSWER
＿＿＿	＿＿＿	Every human cell contains between 50,000 and 100,000 genes.	True. Each cell in the body contains the same genetic information, a code made up of tens of thousands of genes. (See p. 110.)
＿＿＿	＿＿＿	The brain does not exert any control over the immune system.	False. It is believed that the brain can exert control over the immune system, acting as a valuable supplement to conventional medical care. (See p. 58.)
＿＿＿	＿＿＿	The chief role of B cells is the production of antibodies.	True. Every B cell is programmed to make only one specific antibody. (See p. 10.)
＿＿＿	＿＿＿	Asthma is prevalent among West Africans and New Zealand highlanders.	False. In fact, it is rarely reported in these areas, but 3 out of every 100 people in the Western world suffer from this affliction. (See p. 196.)
＿＿＿	＿＿＿	There are 100 trillion cells in the human body.	True. The body is an amazingly complex machine with trillions of cells. (See p. 8.)
＿＿＿	＿＿＿	The size of the thymus gland decreases significantly as a person grows older.	True. The gland weighs about 370 grams at the end of infancy and about 3 grams in old age. (See p. 7.)

UNDERSTANDING
YOUR IMMUNE SYSTEM

chapter 1

Understanding Your Immune System

The terminology used to describe the immune system and its functions sounds much like Defense Department language—and for a good reason. The immune system is exactly like a computerized war machine. It consists of a network of specialized organs and cells whose purpose is to block harmful substances from entering the body and to seek out and destroy those that do invade.

When a baby is born, its defense system is unable to protect it against disease. It has never been exposed to alien invaders such as bacteria and viruses, and so nothing has triggered the manufacture of antibodies. A baby comes into the world with only the antibodies it has received from its mother during gestation. If the baby is breastfed, the mother's milk continues to supply her antibodies to the newborn. During the first weeks of life, the baby's own antibody factories start manufacturing individually designed antibodies that can recognize any substance that is not part of the baby itself. The process continues throughout life, being fine-tuned each successive time the body encounters a foreign substance.

The immune system is a complex network of bodily organs and tissues as well as cellular components that are transported in bodily fluids. It has only been in the last 25 years that scientists have begun to unravel exactly how the immune system operates—and there are still many puzzling aspects of its functioning that remain to be discovered. The system depends on a series of beautifully coordinated cooperative activities that are designed to turn on and off a sequence of immunologic events. Piece by piece, biologists are beginning to sort out and identify the relationship of the various parts to one another and to learn in detail how each one functions.

Many parts of the body are involved in the immune system. It includes the marrow in the long bones, the thymus gland, the spleen, the lymph nodes and their drainage system, the tonsils, the adenoids, and lymphoid tissue in the small intestine called Peyer's patches. Also involved is the reticuloendothelial system, which includes the macrophages lining, the lymph sinuses, and the blood sinuses of the liver, spleen and bone marrow. Some scientists suspect that the appendix may have some role in the immune system as well.

The series of events that involves the immune defense system in our bodies starts before birth, when simple, primitive lymphocytes, which are immature white blood cells, are produced in the bone marrow of the arms, legs, vertebrae, and pelvis. Some of these lymphocytes appear to mature, after birth, either in the bone marrow or in lymph tissue. Others of these white cells, known as stem cells, migrate to the thymus gland. The cells that are aligned with the bone marrow are known as B cells; those that are involved with the thymus are known as T cells. Each of these two types of cells has an individual and specific function.

In very simple terms, the T cells can be described as the infantry of the immune system. They have the ability to kill other cells upon direct contact. The B cells, on the other hand, can be characterized as the artillery, for they discharge bullets known as antibodies, which are designed to recognize unfriendly cells. The B and T cells are organized like no other defense force in the world, because each individual cell is designed to recognize only a single type of alien cell. But when it encounters and recognizes the alien target, the cell starts multiplying. Recognition occurs through binding of the target to specific surface receptors on the defending cell, which brings about a sequence that causes an army of identical clones to be produced.

So well coordinated is a perfectly functioning immune system that it is able to dispense with many invaders in a matter of seconds, and with others—like those that cause colds, influenza, measles, or mumps—within a matter of a few days, usually without serious complications or side effects. It kills off bacterial infections caused by streptococci, pneumococci, and whooping cough and chicken pox. It carries on a lifelong, continuing battle against the hundreds of strains of germs that can cause lingering infections in every part of the body. Through its ability to remember every infection it has ever encountered, it is able to give cradle-to-grave protection against future invasions.

The recognizable outward effects of the immune system in action include a feverish feeling, swollen lymph nodes, weakness, inflammation, diarrhea, nausea, or vomiting—which occur as the various components swing into action and accomplish their goal of killing and removing the offending enemies. When their job is done, the antibodies are depleted and the body returns to normal; we start to feel better, appetite improves, strength returns, and inflammation and swelling lessen and disappear.

Anatomical Participants:
Lymph Nodes, Thymus, Spleen, Bone Marrow, Tonsils, Adenoids, Appendix, Peyer's Patches

What parts of the body are involved in the immune system? This very complex system, many of whose mechanisms are still not fully understood, is made up of the lymph system (lymph nodes and their connecting network of lymphatic channels), the bone marrow, the thymus, the spleen, the tonsils, the appendix, and lymphoid tissue in the small intestine known as Peyer's patches. The various body parts that comprise the immune system are linked with one another by blood vessels and lymph channels. Also included in the functioning of the immune system is the reticuloendothelial system, which serves as an important bodily defense mechanism.

There are an astonishing number of microorganisms in the human colon. Nearly 1 million bacteria are found in each milliliter (.034 fluid ounce) of contents of the intestines—more than 400 different species!

The intestine is sterile at birth. The bacteria come within the first few days of life, picked up at feedings. The organisms help to fight off disease-causing bacteria. Animals delivered by cesarean section and fed sterilized food are not as resistant to disease as those raised in atmospheres that are not free of germs.

Organs of the Immune System

Tonsils and adenoids: Masses of lymphoid tissues in mouth and throat.

Thymus: Source of T cells (killer lymphocytes). Shrinks in size after puberty.

Lymph nodes: Produce lymphocytes. Located in many parts of body. Connected by lymph channels. Nodes vary in size from pinpoint to an inch or so in diameter.

Spleen: Lymphatic organ. Processes lymphocytes and monocytes. Acts as a blood filter.

Peyer's patches: Lymphoid tissue in lower intestine (ileum).

Appendix: Believed to be part of immune system.

Bone marrow: Primitive lymphocytes are produced here in unborn fetus. Source of B cells.

What is the lymph system?

The lymph system works hand in hand with the blood circulatory system but operates with its own subsidiary set of vessels and organs. It performs a number of widely varying jobs. Its primary function is as a drainage network that picks up materials released by body tissues and transports them to the bloodstream. In addition, it is a mainstay of the body's defense system, isolating and neutralizing disease agents. The lymph system absorbs fluid surrounding tissue cells and carries it through ever-larger vessels to each side of the neck, where connections to veins dump the fluid into the bloodstream. The lymph system is also the collecting network for disease-combating white blood cells produced by the bone marrow, thymus, spleen, and tonsils. It produces white cells of its own in the lymph nodes.

Lymph and Blood Systems

Lymph and blood systems are separate but designed to work together. Fluid enters the lymph system from tissue space around lymph capillaries. Vessels returning lymph to blood are interlaced with blood vessels but connect directly only with veins in the neck.

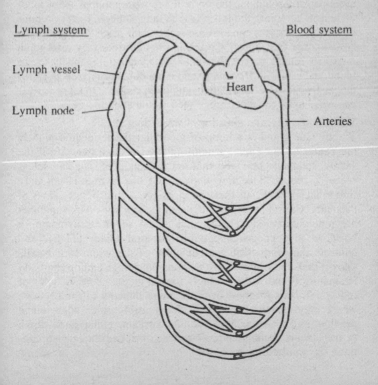

Lymph system

Lymph vessel

Lymph node

Heart

Blood system

Arteries

What do lymph nodes do?

Lymph nodes are small bean-shaped structures that hang in neck-lacelike strings throughout the body. Strings of lymph nodes are found in the neck, armpits, abdomen, and groin. Each individual bean-shaped node contains a variety of specialized compartments; these compartments separately house B cells, T cells, and macrophages. The nodes also contain webbed areas that trap and filter out foreign substances (antigens). The nodes are linked by the network of lymphatic vessels, which are similar in structure to blood vessels and function as a drainage system.

The lymphatic vessels drain from every part of the body. They come together at the base of the neck and empty into the bloodstream. Via the lymphatic vessels, lymphocytes and other assorted cells of the immune system are carried to the bloodstream, which delivers them to tissues throughout the body. The lymphocytes patrol throughout the body for foreign antigens, then gradually drift back into the lymphatic system to begin the cycle once more. Lymphocytes can also remember their place of origin. Thus lymphocytes from Peyer's patch in the intestines may react to an intestinal infection, circulate through lymphatic channels to the blood and return to Peyer's patch. This circulatory path is called the gastrointestinal associated lymphatic tissue (GALT). Similar pathways exist for other areas such as the skin and eyes.

What is the thymus gland and what does it do?

The thymus gland is a lump of glandular tissue located high in the center of the chest, straddling the tracheal area. Until the 1960s, scientists believed that the thymus gland was a useless piece of tissue. It is now known that the thymus is not only important but can, in fact, be considered the master gland of the body's immune system even though many of its functions are not understood. The thymus gland secretes thymosin—a hormone also known as thymic humoral factor (THF)—and controls the production and function of the white blood cells known as T cells, which are responsible for defending the body against viral and fungal infections and against certain types of tumors. T cells migrate from the bone marrow to the thymus, where they remain for a time and multiply; then some leave the thymus and, by way of the bloodstream, either settle down in the spleen, tonsils, lymph nodes, or appendix or else continue to circulate in the blood.

What happens to the thymus as it ages?

In the first 3 months of life, infants have fragile, incomplete immune systems. However, their thymus glands are busy producing a supply of T cells that will be able to mount defenses against infection. At the end of this period, the thymus weighs about 370 grams. After puberty, it appears to begin to shrink, and in the elderly it weighs about 3 grams. In effect, then, the thymus gland reaches its greatest relative weight at birth, increases in weight until about the age of 14, when the body achieves puberty. Thereafter it begins to decrease in weight, and much of the lymphoid tissue is replaced by fat. Though reduced in size, the thymus does continue to have some effect on the immune system even late in life.

What is the role of the spleen in the immune system?

The spleen is a large lymph-nodelike but ductless organ located in the upper part of the abdominal cavity on the left side. It has a flattened oblong shape and is the largest structure in the immune system. Its functions, though not completely understood, include disintegrating the red blood cells and setting free hemoglobin, producing new red blood cells during fetal life and in the newborn, serving as a reservoir of blood, and producing lymphocytes and plasma cells. Circulating lymphocytes may spend several hours in the spleen. Persons whose spleens have been damaged by accident or by disease can be quite susceptible to infection. Once removed, the spleen does not grow back, but many of its functions appear to be taken over by other body tissues.

What is the function of the bone marrow in the immune system?

The bone marrow, the soft tissue in the hollow shafts of the long bones, produces white cells, which are an important part of the immune response system.

What roles do the tonsils, adenoids, appendix, and Peyer's patches play in the immune system?

Each of these have heavy concentrations of lymphoid tissue. Though their specific roles in immune defense are not completely documented, it is known that these closely packed collections of lymphoid nodules act as special sentinels in the specific part of the body where each is located.

Cellular Participants:
B Cells, T Cells, Lymphokines, Granulocytes, Natural Killer Cells, Macrophages, Monocytes, Monokines

How many cells are there in the human body?

There are 100 trillion cells in the human body—100,000,-000,000,000. The cells, as needed, make copies of themselves. That happens billions of times during the course of a person's life. In any given second, some 20 million cells in your body are dividing . . . with each one becoming two cells.

What are the different kinds of cells produced by the immune system?

The immune system has a tremendous stockpile of cells that perform a wide variety of functions. The cells are white cells, as distinguished from the red cells also seen in blood under the microscope. There are many different types, and defining them is made all the more confusing because some types are known by a number of different names. *Leukocyte,* for example, which is a general overall name for all white cells, is sometimes spelled *leucocyte* and can also be mistakenly referred to as a macrophage, a phagocyte, a polymorphonuclear leukocyte, or a polymorph. Lymphocytes are leukocytes that are found mostly in the lymphoid tissues. They fall into two categories: B cells (cells that are produced in the bone marrow) and T cells (cells that are primarily formed in the thymus). Another type of leukocyte is known as a phagocyte, meaning that it is a scavenger cell. These come in three varieties: macrophages, the garbage collectors that usually present antigens to the T cells; monocytes, which circulate through the blood, engulfing and digesting antigen particles; and granulocytes, some of which are called natural killer cells, containing granules filled with potent chemicals that enable them to digest microorganisms. These granulocyte chemicals also contribute to inflammatory reactions and are responsible for the symptoms of allergy.

Cell Types Organization Chart

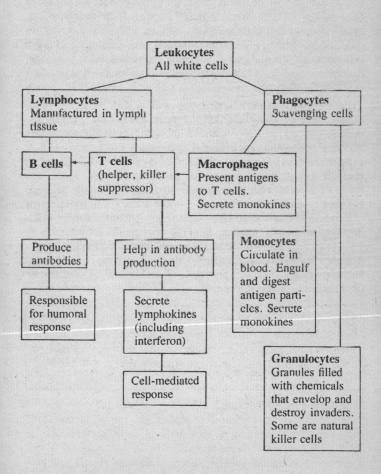

What is the role of B cells?

B cells produce the antibodies required to combat invading antigens. Each B cell is programmed to make only one specific antibody, which will combine with its corresponding antigen in lock-and-key fashion. When a B cell encounters its matching antigen, it matures into plasma cells, which are individual factories for producing antibodies. Each plasma cell derived from a given B cell manufactures millions of antibody molecules, each producing the same antibody, which it releases into the bloodstream.

What do T cells do?

T cells come in a variety of types with a wide range of functions—many of which are still not fully understood even by the most knowledgeable biologists. Although T cells do not secrete antibodies, their help is essential in antibody production. *Helper T cells* bolster the activity of B cells. *Suppressor T cells* act to shut off that activity when it has gone far enough. These two types of T cells keep the immune defense system in balance. Another type of T cells, known as *killer T cells,* can be activated to become killers themselves—destroying bacteria, cancer cells, or cells infected by viruses. Some T cells produce *lymphokines,* which can help bring other immune cells into action in the body's defense. Unlike B cells, which can recognize and attack free-floating viruses or other particles, T cells seem to concentrate their action exclusively on cells.

Every minute, it is estimated, some 300 million cells die in the body, most of them to be replaced immediately by the division of the cells that remain, so that the total number of cells in the adult body remains virtually constant throughout life.

What are T-cell receptors?

T-cell receptors are chemical configurations on the surface of T cells that act as keys in a lock-and-key identification system. Until 1984, scientists were unable to figure out how the T cell was able to recognize invading enemies such as viruses and bacteria. Common sense told them that there must be some sort of recognition receptor on the surface of the cell, but no one was able to determine the chemical and physical structure of the receptor and its genes. The search came to an end when two teams of scientists, almost simultaneously, independently identified the T-cell receptors. This discovery opens the way for more research, which may soon unlock the entire chain of events that triggers the actions of T cells.

What are lymphokines?

Lymphokines are the potent chemical secretions that mobilize the body's defenses. These neurotransmitters, of which there are about fifty different types, are produced in infinitesimal quantities by T cells. Lymphokines fit in lock-and-key fashion to receptors on other types of white cells. Until recently, large amounts of human blood were required to isolate a tiny sample of lymphokines. Genetic engineering has now made it possible for scientists to isolate and produce large quantities of lymphokines outside the human body.

Two of the lymphokines, gamma interferon and interleukin 2, are being tested for clinical application. Interleukin 2 appears to be the key lymphokine, the one that serves as the primary signal to activate the immune system, causing T cells to proliferate. Gamma interferon kills cancer cells, prevents viruses from invading cells, and enhances the activity of killer cells and macrophages.

Other lymphokines that have been isolated and are being tested include colony stimulating factor (CSF), which causes the bone marrow to produce lymphocytes; macrophage activating factor (MAF), which stimulates macrophages to seek out and ingest invading organisms and cancer cells; and B-cell growth factor (BCGF), which triggers B cells to divide and begin producing antibodies.

What happens to the B and T cells when they age?

Marguerite B. Kay, a medical researcher at Texas A & M University, has found that old cells literally commit suicide by triggering the immune system to destroy them and remove them from the body. When a cell reaches the end of its life span, it produces an antigen on its surface that binds to an antibody that is always circulating in the bloodstream. Scavenging macrophages then ingest and destroy the old cells.

What is a granulocyte?

Granulocytes are white cells filled with granules of toxic chemicals that enable them to digest microorganisms. The granulocytes that attack and destroy tumor cells and those infected with viruses or other microbes are sometimes referred to as natural killer, or NK, cells. Basophils, neutrophils, eosinophils, and mast cells are other types of granulocytes. The chemicals in granulocytes also contribute to inflammatory reactions and are responsible for the symptoms of allergy.

What are natural killer cells?
Natural killer cells are granulocytes that attack and destroy other cells. They are known as natural killers because they strike without prior stimulation by a specific antigen. Tumor cells, as well as normal cells infected with a virus, are susceptible to the natural

---

The immune system is so effective that it can destroy an incompatible transplanted kidney in 10 days.

---

killer cells. Normal cells are resistant to the activity of natural killer cells. Biologists believe that natural killer cells play a key role in preventing cancer in the healthy body, since they hunt down cells that develop abnormal changes and kill them before they can start doing damage.

What are macrophages and monocytes?
Like granulocytes, macrophages and monocytes are capable of enveloping and destroying invaders. Monocytes circulate freely in the blood, while macrophages are found in body tissues, some macrophages also play a critical role in initiating immune response by presenting antigens to T cells in a special way that allows the T cells to recognize them. Macrophages and monocytes secrete an array of powerful chemical substances, called monokines, which help to direct and regulate the immune response.

What are monokines?
Monokines are powerful chemical substances secreted by macrophages and monocytes. They are comparable to the lymphokines secreted by lymphocytes. Like lymphokines, monokines help to direct and regulate the immune response. Interleukin 1 is a monokine which triggers healing of injuries. Because it also causes inflammation and fever, it is believed to play a role in chronic inflammatory diseases such as rheumatoid arthritis.

Functions of Immune System: B Cells and T Cells are Separate but Interlocking

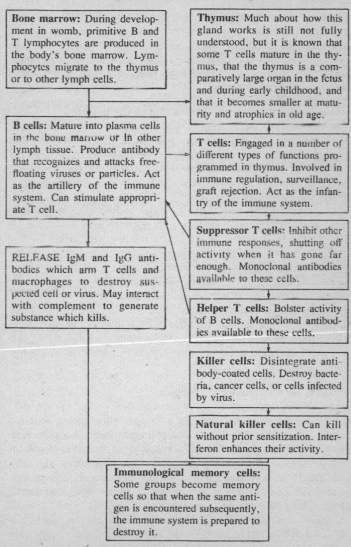

Bone marrow: During development in womb, primitive B and T lymphocytes are produced in the body's bone marrow. Lymphocytes migrate to the thymus or to other lymph cells.

Thymus: Much about how this gland works is still not fully understood, but it is known that some T cells mature in the thymus, that the thymus is a comparatively large organ in the fetus and during early childhood, and that it becomes smaller at maturity and atrophies in old age.

B cells: Mature into plasma cells in the bone marrow or in other lymph tissue. Produce antibody that recognizes and attacks free-floating viruses or particles. Act as the artillery of the immune system. Can stimulate appropriate T cell.

T cells: Engaged in a number of different types of functions programmed in thymus. Involved in immune regulation, surveillance, graft rejection. Act as the infantry of the immune system.

**RELEASE IgM and IgG antibodies which arm T cells and macrophages to destroy suspected cell or virus. May interact with complement to generate substance which kills.

Suppressor T cells: Inhibit other immune responses, shutting off activity when it has gone far enough. Monoclonal antibodies available to these cells.

Helper T cells: Bolster activity of B cells. Monoclonal antibodies available to these cells.

Killer cells: Disintegrate antibody-coated cells. Destroy bacteria, cancer cells, or cells infected by virus.

Natural killer cells: Can kill without prior sensitization. Interferon enhances their activity.

Immunological memory cells: Some groups become memory cells so that when the same antigen is encountered subsequently, the immune system is prepared to destroy it.

Antigens, Antibodies, Immune Response

What are antigens?
Antigens are substances that are foreign to the body and can therefore trigger an immune response. An antigen can be a virus, a bacterium, a fungus, or a parasite—any organism that the body's natural response rejects. Tissues or cells from one person's body can act as antigens when transplanted or transfused to the body of another person.

What happens when an antigen enters the body?
The immune system is full of interlocking and overlapping systems with checks and balances and cooperative activities that produce similar end results and are designed to turn on or off a sequence of immunologic events. To fend off the hordes of bacteria, viruses, parasites, and fungi that threaten the system, the body has a choreographed series of defenses. To enter, microbes must first find a chink in the body's external protection. The mucous membranes are coated with antibodies, which can immediately decimate and carry off invaders. Various microbes will be intercepted by patrolling scavenger cells. Then, if they escape these traps, the body's more specific responses are called into action. These include *cellular responses,* directed by cells—especially T cells and their secretions—or *humoral responses,* which are performed by antibodies that have been secreted by B cells into the body's fluids. The two parts of the immune system, cellular and humoral, are closely allied, and most invading antigens stimulate both a cellular and a humoral response.

What is the complement system?
The complement system is made up of a series of approximately 20 proteins that circulate in the blood in an inactive form. When the first of the complement substances is triggered—usually by an antibody locked to an antigen—it sets in motion what is known as the complement cascade. As each component is activated, like a pebble in a pond, it sets into action the next in a precise sequence of carefully regulated steps. This complement cascade is responsible for causing cells to release the chemicals that produce the redness, warmth, and swelling of the inflammatory response. Complement is also able

to punch a hole in the cell wall of an invader and thus destroy it. (This process is known as lysis.)

How is the immune system able to recognize the many different antigens?

By storing just a few cells specific for each potential invader, the body is able to protect itself against all its enemies. When an antigen appears, the specially designed antibodies are stimulated to multiply.

How many antibodies are there?

It is estimated that the body makes a total of more than 10 million different kinds of antibodies. One or another of these almost always matches an identifying chemical structure, called an antigen, on any substance foreign to the body.

How do antibodies work?

Antibodies circulate freely in body fluids. Some disable the toxins produced by bacteria, or block viruses from entering into healthy cells. Some have the ability to activate the complement cascade that will kill the cell and signal scavenger cells to destroy and carry them away. Antibodies cannot penetrate living cells and are therefore ineffective against microorganisms inside cells.

Where are antibodies manufactured?

B cells secrete antibodies. Every B cell is programmed to make only one specific antibody.

How are antibodies identified?

There are five classes of antibodies, also known as immunoglobulins. All are classified by the prefix *Ig*, which is an abbreviation for *immunoglobulin*. The prefix is then followed by the letters *G*, *A*, *M*, *D*, or *E*. Each class of antibodies plays a different role. IgG, the major immunoglobulin in the blood, is also able to enter tissue spaces. It works efficiently to coat microorganisms, speeding their uptake by other cells in the immune system. IgM, which usually combines in star-shaped clusters, tends to remain in the bloodstream, where it is very effective at killing bacteria. IgA concentrates in body fluids like tears and saliva, as well as in the secretions of the respiratory and gastrointestinal tracts, guarding the entrances to the body. IgE attaches itself to the surface of the specialized immune cells such as mast cells and basophils and, when it encounters its matching antigen, stimulates the specialized cell to pour out its contents. IgD is almost exclusively inserted into cell membranes, where it somehow regulates the activation of the cell.

Is there a different antibody for each disease?

Yes. The system is amazingly specific. The antibody that is produced against mumps will attack the mumps virus and nothing else. That means that the immune system is able to turn out millions of different kinds of antibodies—each one as a specific reaction against one substance.

Is a person forever immune to a particular disease once he or she has recovered from it?

Once the immune system counterattacks with antibodies and the army of antibodies has been activated against a particular invader, the antibodies continue to circulate for years afterward. If you have had a bout with mumps, for instance, you will be immune to mumps for many years.

How does the body remember what diseases it has been exposed to?

Whenever T cells and B cells are activated, some groups become memory cells so that when an individual encounters the same antigen again, the immune system is prepared to destroy it. The degree of immunity depends on the kind of antigen, its amount, and how it enters the body.

What is natural immunity?

Natural immunity is the protection we inherit from our mothers at birth, and which is built into our immune system. Infants are born with relatively weak immune responses, though they are protected during the first months of life by means of antibodies they receive from their mothers before birth. The antibody IgG, which travels across the placenta, makes them immune to the same microbes to which their mothers are immune. Infants who are nursed also receive additional immunity through IgA antibodies in breast milk.

What Happens When the Body Goes into Action Against an Ordinary Invader Such as a Virus

Virus enters body, attaches to cell membrane, comes out of its protein coat, and releases its DNA and/or RNA into host cell and begins to replicate. ⟶ Cell responds by releasing certain lymphokines and monokines. T and B cells are alerted that danger is in the area.

Low-grade fever may result at this point. ⟶ Cells challenge and test invader. Demand password. Recognize foreignness. Take note of surface markers. Report to nearest lymph-node headquarters.

Local swelling of lymph nodes and increased white blood count. ⟶ T cells kill on contact if possible or report to thymus, which instructs lymph nodes to release T lymphocytes sensitized to invader. Meanwhile, B lymphocytes release IgM, then IgG antibodies, which have several areas that attach themselves to invader.

Causes increased serum complement. ⟶ This action triggers change in antibody shape, which activates complement cascade—molecules and special proteins in bloodstream capable of neutralizing or destroying invaders.

Lack of appetite, weakness, inflammation, generalized aches and pains. ⟶ Antigens pour into bloodstream. Antibodies attach themselves to surface markers of invaders, causing them to clump together.

Diarrhea, nausea, vomiting, and inflammation. ⟶ Histamine and other chemicals are released, which stimulate macrophages.

Improved appetite, decreased fatigue and inflammation, lowered blood-cell counts. ⟶ Macrophages ingest dead tissue and injured cells and dispose of them.

Some cells return to lymph tissue, where they remain dormant until invader appears again. They "remember" the invader and provide future rapid response and long-term immunity.

What is acquired immunity?

When vaccines containing microorganisms or parts of microorganisms are used to stimulate the body to produce antibodies against specific diseases, the body is forced to take the necessary steps to acquire immunity against the disease. This type of immunity is known as acquired immunity.

Can a baby survive if it is born lacking an immune defense system?

Such a condition is known as severe combined immunodeficiency disease (SCID). Some children with SCID have lived for many years in germ-free rooms and "bubbles." Some experimental work has been done in treating a few SCID patients with transplants of bone marrow. This treatment has been successful in converting the immature cells in the bone-marrow transplant into functioning B and T cells.

Does the body sometimes make errors in identifying antigens?

Autoimmune diseases or diseases of immune regulation result when the body makes a mistake—that is, when the body wrongly identifies self as nonself. Rheumatoid arthritis and systemic lupus are examples of diseases that result from errors in the immune computer. Similarly, allergies are caused by an improper response of the immune system to a harmless substance such as ragweed or dust.

What are the various kinds of disorders of the immune system?

With so complex a system, the possibilities for error or miscalculation are great, spanning a wide spectrum of problems. Lack of one or more components of the immune system results in an *immune deficiency* disease. When cells grow uncontrollably, *immunoproliferative* disorders result. When the balance of the cells is at fault, disorders of *immune regulation* are seen. *Immune complex* diseases occur when clusters of interlocking antigens and antibodies are not properly removed from the body. *Autoimmune diseases* are seen when the body manufactures antibodies directed against itself. And, of course, *allergies* are the result of the immune system responding to a false alarm.

What factors can cause malfunctioning of the immune system?

The immune system may work improperly when there is a lack

of one or more components of the immune system. This can be an inherited condition, or it can result from common viral infections such as flu, mononucleosis, or measles. Immune system malfunction can also be caused by the side effects of some drug treatments or blood transfusions, as well as by anesthesia. Malnutrition, stress, and environmental factors also play a role.

How Strong Is Your Immune System?

	Your Answer		Scoring		Your Score
	Yes	No	Yes	No	
I come from a family with strong genes: At least one parent and one grandparent lived to be 80 or older.			+1	—	
I was breastfed for a month or more.			+1	—	
I have never had anesthesia.			+1	—	
I have had a serious injury during the past 2 years.			—	+1	
I have had mononucleosis.			—	+1	
I have had my spleen removed.			—	+1	
I am over age 50.			—	+1	
I am cautious about having X rays.			+1	—	
I am between 10 and 19 or over 50 and have had X rays in the last year.			—	+1	
I allow myself to get overtired often.			—	+1	
I am under constant stress.			—	+1	
I have a positive attitude and consider myself very healthy.			+1	—	
I have a good self-image.			+1	—	
I have good long-term relationships with people.			+1	—	
I feel hostile toward many people.			—	+1	
I have loving, caring people in my life.			+1	—	
I eat a healthy, nourishing diet.			+1	—	
I eat a lot of meat, dairy products, ice cream, fried foods, salty snacks.			—	+1	
I eat foods that are steamed, boiled, stewed, baked.			+1	—	
I prefer charcoal-broiled or grilled meats.			—	+1	
I am often constipated.			—	+1	
I supplement my diet with vitamins.			+1	—	
I take vitamin C supplements.			+1	—	
I am a smoker.			—	+1	

20

	Your Answer		Scoring		Your Score
	Yes	No	Yes	No	
I probably drink too much alcohol.		✗	—	+1	
I spend a lot of time in the sun.		✗	—	+1	
I get some exercise daily.	✗		+1	—	
I never seem to be able to relax.		✗	—	+1	
I often feel helpless to change things.		✗	—	+1	
I get plenty of grains and fiber in my diet.	✗		+1	—	
I eat lots of green and yellow vegetables.	✗		+1	—	
I get lots of colds.		✗	—	+1	
I had the flu this year.		✗	—	+1	
I have allergies.		✗	—	+1	
I feel in control of my job and my life.	✗		+1	—	
I feel change is a challenge rather than a threat.	✗		+1	—	

30–35   You are doing very well. Keep up your good habits.
20–30   You are on your way. Take a look at some of those personal habits that you can change.
Under 20 You need to look seriously at your lifestyle and start making some changes.

chapter 2

Where the Problems Are

Immune systems vary considerably in effectiveness from one individual to another. To some extent this difference is a matter of inheritance, which determines the quality of the immunological defense system with which we are born.

Other factors are also involved. Aging is the most apparent. As we age, not only is it increasingly difficult for us to fight off disease, but it seems that all our systems are geared to a decline in function. Scientists ponder whether the aging phenomenon is tied to the chance mutation of ordinary cells—or whether our entire mechanism is programmed to self-destruct. With age, our cells progressively fail to reproduce themselves properly, copying genetic instructions with more and more errors. At the same time, the body has been increasingly exposed to a variety of lifestyle and environmental factors that also cause cells to make mistakes. In the normal course of events, the healthy immune system destroys cell mutations. When this normal action weakens, the damaging effects on tissues of the body increase the speed of aging, and multiply the possibilities of allowing immune disorders. Tests of people over 65 show that although they can still produce antibody at the normal rate to combat any antigen they are known to have encountered in their younger days, most are very slow at, and some actually incapable of, producing antibody against an unknown or unusual invader.

When all the life events that appear to contribute to the weakening of the normal immune system are considered in addition to the normal aging phenomenon, the possibilities for immune problems become monumental. A host of factors have been studied, and many have been found to have a profound bearing on what happens to the functioning of the immune cells. The list includes stress, lifestyle habits, surgery, anesthesia, and pain, as well as environmental factors such as carcinogens and mutagens found in everyday life.

Factors within our control, and factors over which we have no control, are involved. Though our immune systems are imprinted before we are born, and strengthened again in the early weeks of life by breastfeeding, they evolve daily as the 100 trillion cells that make up our bodies undergo change. It is evident that we can't blame all the weaknesses or strengths of our immune systems on our ancestors. We must look closely at the other factors involved, recognize the possible problems, and learn how we can do something about them.

Aging

What changes in the organs of the immune system are associated with aging?

The most dramatic changes from birth to old age occur in the thymus gland. It starts to shrink after sexual maturity and continues to shrivel until, by the age of 45 or 50, it is only 5 to 10 percent of its weight at puberty. Since it serves both as a site of cellular activity and as the master gland of the immune system, these changes have a significant effect on the way the system functions in old age. The movement of immature lymphocytes from bone marrow to thymus decreases. Several hormones synthesized in the thymus begin to decrease between ages 20 and 30, completely disappearing by the time normal humans are over 60 years of age.

What changes occur in the functioning of lymphocytes as we age?

Fewer immature lymphocytes enter the thymus with age, and the ratio of immature lymphocytes to other lymphocytes within the thymus and the blood increases with age, suggesting that the aging thymus gland loses its capacity to process immature lymphocytes. Although the number of T and B lymphocytes does not seem to change with age, there is a decrease of them in the lymph nodes and an increase in the plasma cells. And though their total numbers are the same, their capacity for immune response is not.

Does age cause a change in immunoglobulin levels?

The concentration of immunoglobulins changes little with age, but the distribution of the various types of immunoglobulins does change. The concentration of IgA and IgG (which make up more than 90 percent of the immunoglobulins in normal blood) increases, and the concentration of the other immunoglobulins decreases.

Is there a change in the number of antibodies as we grow older?

Yes. The number of antibodies decreases. However, the number of autoantibodies (antibodies that attack our own cells) increases. Even with the increase in autoantibodies, autoimmune diseases such as lupus and rheumatoid arthritis do not occur with greater frequency in the elderly.

Does aging affect the immune system, or does the immune system affect aging?

It's a chicken-and-egg question—and one that is being widely discussed. In animal studies there is a great deal of evidence that aging affects the immune system. In humans it is not as clear which is the cause and which is the effect. Diseases such as cancer, which are more prevalent in the aging population, may be caused by a breakdown in the immune system. Interestingly, however, diseases most involved with autoantibodies and connective tissues, such as lupus and rheumatoid arthritis, are not confined to older age groups and are more common in women than in men.

Does aging affect everyone's immune system the same way?

A great deal of research is being done on the topic of aging and the immune system. Much of it is focused on the question of why people age differently. Mice studies show that cells age differently in different strains of mice. Age-dependent changes in thymus gland activity, in B cells, and in suppressor T cells also vary among different strains. The ages at which the cells are not as resistant to foreign substances differ, as do the changes in metabolism. Researchers feel that there must be genetic controls in some of the age-related changes and that not all of these are due to an accumulation of life events. Much more research is needed in analyzing both the cellular and the genetic causes of aging to discover those markers that will allow doctors to predict persons at risk for aging disorders.

What are the effects of potassium deficiency on aging?

Researchers believe that cellular leakage of potassium may contribute to cell aging, which can in effect contribute to increasing cancer rates in older people. Research has shown that a characteristic occurrence of aging is an inflow of sodium into the cells and a corresponding reduction of potassium and eventual excretion of potassium from the body.

What is Werner's syndrome?

Werner's syndrome, a disease that prematurely ages young children, is characterized by senility, graying and loss of hair, cataracts, skin changes, and an impaired immune system. Researchers hope that study of this disease will yield clues to aging questions.

Can the aging process in the human body be slowed down in the same way that chemical preservatives retard the aging of food?

It's possible that the chemicals that preserve food preserve us too. Though preservatives have been under attack by consumer groups, antioxidants (chemicals that delay or prevent foods from becoming old, stale, or rancid) appear to have a similar effect on humans. Chemicals such as BHT, BHA, propyl gallate, and TBHQ have been used since World War II by American food producers to prolong food life. It is possible, though it has not been proven scientifically, that the decrease in stomach cancer in the United States may be somehow attributable to the widespread use of these antioxidants. In Japan, where antioxidants are not used regularly in food preservation, stomach cancer is on the increase. This controversial subject has led some health proponents to add BHT supplements to their diets in an attempt to preserve the body in much the same way that foods are preserved.

Stress

What kinds of stresses put a strain on the body?

Many things cause stress. Any kind of tissue injury, general infections, excessive fatigue, exposure to heat or cold, an operation, anesthesia, or medication put extra stress on the body. Stressors range from emotions to malnutrition. Stressful situations are not always unpleasant and include such commonplace activities as a game of football or strenuous physical exercise. Even a passionate kiss can produce stress. Researchers are now classifying stress into different categories. For instance, they feel that the body reacts differently to normal stress that has become a chronic occurrence than to pleasant stress, such as when you've worked hard and are happy about a successful accomplishment.

What is the hypothalamus?

The hypothalamus acts as the thermostat of the brain. A tiny cluster of nerve cells at the base of the brain, its function is to integrate and ensure appropriate responses to stimuli. It receives impulses of messages from both the conscious and subconscious parts of the brain and then sends out signals via both nerves and hormones.

What is the pituitary gland, and what does it do?

The pituitary gland is a pea-sized organ that is linked to the hypothalamus by a short, stubby stalk. It hangs from the undercarriage of the brain in a small bony hollow, behind the nose and between the eyes. It is separated into two lobes, which secrete numerous hormones which have a wide range of effects upon the growth, metabolism, and other functions of the body. These hormones include:

- Growth hormone (GH);
- Prolactin, which stimulates milk secretions;
- Thyroid-stimulating hormone (TSH) or thyrotroph, which stimulates thyroid growth and secretion;
- Adrenocorticotrophic hormone (ACTH), which stimulates the adrenal cortex, an energy-generating gland;
- Follicle-stimulating hormone (FSH), which stimulates ovarian follicle growth in the female and sperm production in the male;
- Luteinizing hormone (LH), which provokes ovulation in the female and stimulates release of the sex hormone testosterone in the male;
- Oxytocin, which causes contraction of the uterus during pregnancy and acts on certain muscle cells that control milk during nursing;
- Vasopressin, which acts on kidney tubes to regulate body fluid, sodium and potassium concentrations;
- Melanocyte-stimulating hormone (MSH), which controls skin pigment.

Where are the adrenal glands located, and what do they do?
The adrenal glands sit perched like a three-cornered hat on the upper surface of each kidney. Each gland is really a gland within a gland, consisting of a pea-sized central core known as the adrenal medulla and a thicker outer surface, the adrenal cortex.

The medulla releases epinephrine (adrenaline) as well as smaller quantities of norepinephrine (noradrenaline), a closely related substance. If epinephrine is injected into the body, a complex series of physiological changes occurs. The blood pressure is elevated, arteries constrict, blood sugar levels rise, cardiac output is increased, blood vessels dilate, and, if animal tests are valid, the spleen contracts, ejecting the stored blood cells into the bloodstream. The body is mobilized for unusual exertion. This response is known as the fight-or-flight reaction.

The adrenal cortex is an endocrine factory secreting many hormonelike materials. About fifty of them have been identified so far, of which ten are very active. Although all the hormones have the same basic chemical structure (and are called adrenocorticosteroids), each has a strikingly different functional purpose, of which there are three categories:

1. Glucocorticoids act primarily in regulating sugar and protein metabolism.
2. Mineralocorticoids regulate the amount of sodium and other minerals in extracellular fluids.
3. Sex hormones control the secondary sex characteristics.

What mechanisms are involved in the body's response to stress?
There are chain reactions involved in the body's response to stress. The brain, by interpreting an event as psychologically threatening, begins the chain by sending a message to the hypothalamus, whose main job is to regulate essential life-support systems. The hypothalamus stimulates release of a substance that directs the pituitary gland to make ACTH, a hormone that stimulates the adrenal cortex to release corticosteroids. Corticosteroids are chemical compounds that usually function to reduce inflammation but can also, under prolonged stress, suppress the immune system. The pituitary gland can also signal the release of endorphins, which are natural painkillers for the body.

A similar chain reaction can begin when the hypothalamus

relays a message to the adrenal medulla to trigger the release of eight other hormones. Epinephrine triggers the release of sugar stored in the liver, makes the heart beat more quickly, quickens breathing, and makes the blood flow away from the skin and digestive system and toward the brain and skeletal muscles. The thymus gland, which produces infection-fighting white blood cells, is shrunk by corticosteroids. Some of the hormones released during the stress response suppress the immune system, while others stimulate it. The exact workings of all these mechanisms are still being researched.

How do stress messages get from the brain to the immune system?
Though the research in this area is in its infancy, it seems that there may be two paths: one from the brain to endocrine gland to lymphocytes, and the other from the brain via nerve endings to lymphocytes. A number of researchers have found that lymphocytes have receptors for chemicals such as those released during response to stress (adrenaline and noradrenaline). It is thought that these may help regulate the immune system.

> At Harvard Medical School, immunologists looking for the chemical mechanism by which the brain controls the immune system found that when the lymphocyte cells prepare to attack foreign substances, molecular structures called receptors appear on their surfaces. These receptors bind chemically to acetylcholine, one of the main transmitters of signals between the nerves. Even in laboratory dishes, acetylcholine stimulates the lymphocytes to prepare to fight.

Karen Bullock of the State University of New York at Stony Brook and David Felten of the University of Rochester have independently reported finding sympathetic nerve endings in such organs as the lymph nodes and spleen, both of which provide sources of antigens for lymphocytes. The nerve endings are near fields of lymphocytes, with their receptors for norepinephrine. The researchers' theory is that the lymphocytes probably represent a target for the nerve terminals so that the brain may communicate directly with the free-roaming cell populations.

Stress Alters Functions of Many Glands and Organs

Brain interprets an event as threatening.

Hypothalamus stimulates pituitary gland and sympathetic nervous system.

Pituitary releases hormones, including ACTH and pain-lulling endorphins.

Thymus produces infection-fighting white blood cells. Is shrunk by corticosteroids.

ACTH stimulates adrenal cortex to release corticosteroids, which can suppress immune system.

Adrenal medulla secretes epinephrine and norepinephrine.

Epinephrine appears to bind to receptor sites on surface of white blood cells, inhibiting immune response.

Liver triggers release of stored sugar useful in flight-or-fight response.

Epinephrine and sympathetic nervous system stimulate heartbeat.

Parasympathetic nervous system can cause ulcers.

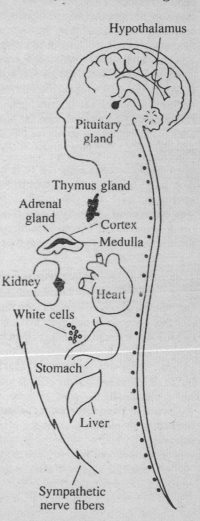

Does the body respond differently to short-term and long-term stresses?

It is now thought that when stress is long term, the adrenal glands secrete cortisol rather than the epinephrine produced in response to short-term stress. Cortisol is a glucocorticoid whose effects are not well understood. What is known is that cortisol acts more slowly than does epinephrine and raises the blood pressure gradually. It makes the small blood vessels more sensitive to epinephrine and, with epinephrine, helps make the platelets (the cells in the blood that work to clot the blood after injury or cut) more sticky, thus making it easier for blood clots to form. Cortisol also represses sex hormones.

How does the body respond to the alleviation of stress?

The hypothalamus, the area of the brain that signals the response to stress to begin, can also signal it to slow down. This was discovered in the 1940s by Swiss Nobel prizewinner Walter B. Hess. Heart rate, breathing, and body metabolism all slow down, and the entire sympathetic nervous system becomes relaxed.

Is there a relationship between illness and stress?

Many studies have indicated a relationship between stressful situations, especially life events, and illness. Diabetes mellitus, heart disease, cirrhosis of the liver, and asthma are recognized as stress-related disorders, but studies increasingly show a much wider range of disorders associated with the experience of stressful events. There are illnesses in which the mechanism by which stress could cause disease is less obvious but which clearly involve the immune system in some way. They range from colds to influenza, from tuberculosis to arthritis and cancer, from lower back pain to recurrent flare-ups of herpes, skin blemishes, and allergies.

Both animal and human studies show that emotional reactions can stimulate or suppress disease-fighting white blood cells and trigger the release of hormones from glands and the nervous system, which in turn can affect many of the body processes. They also show that a person's inability to cope with stress may affect the immune system, causing the white blood cells to lose some of their ability to fight off disease.

What effect does loss of a close family member have on health?

The National Academy of Sciences reports that the death of a close family member leaves some survivors vulnerable to physical or mental illness. Although the researchers noted wide variations in individual responses, they found that patterns of life can be disrupted for at least 1 year or for as long as 3 years.

Bereaved men under the age of 75 run an increased risk of death from some infectious diseases, heart disease, and accidents. Bereaved women's risk of death may rise in the second year, and female survivors show greater relative risk of cirrhosis and possibly suicide. Survivors, both male and female, who have strong social support systems, or who remarry, appear to suffer fewer health problems.

If stress produces illness, how can some people experience many difficult life events and not become ill?

Three factors seem to make a difference: social support, predictability, and control. It has been suggested that an individual who believes he or she is cared for, loved, and esteemed and is surrounded by caring persons can be protected from a wide range of illnesses, including arthritis, tuberculosis, depression, and alcoholism. It has also been indicated that this support can reduce the amount of medication needed and speed recovery. An individual who is able to anticipate what is going to happen and feels some control over the situation generally suffers fewer adverse effects from the event. Researchers believe that a feeling of helplessness usually intensifies stress, whereas a sense of control reduces stress. Stress is also reduced when a person is aware that something is going to happen and is given information about the event. For instance, patients who know that painkillers are available when needed experience less discomfort and need fewer painkillers than those who are restricted to painkillers on a prescribed schedule. Dental surgeons report that patients who have had their treatments described step by step and can stop the treatment at any point with a hand signal are better able to relax and tolerate treatment.

Is it possible that some back problems are connected to stress and the immune system?

Many physicians have concluded that there is a connection between backaches and emotions. Some feel that depression plays a role but do not know whether the depression causes the back pain or the back pain causes the depression. Others feel that tension and emotions can make blood vessels constrict, thereby interfering with oxygen supplies to some muscles and nerves, which results in the sensation of pain. The fear that comes with the first sharp pain causes more pain. Learning how to relax and doing exercises to deal with stress has helped many people who suffer from backaches.

Is there a connection between stress and viral diseases?

In general, it would appear that stress increases susceptibility to a variety of infectious agents. Studies have been performed on animals inoculated with various viruses and "stressed" in different ways—either with light and electric shock or with restraint plus food and water deprivation. In most experiments, the animals who died came from the "stressed" groups; autopsies revealed that these animals also had greater amounts of virus present in various organs.

There were some differences, mostly based on when the inoculations were given in comparison with the stress. All studies did not show that stressed animals were more susceptible, however. In a few studies there were no differences in susceptibility; in others, the stressed animals were less susceptible. Age, sex, and type of animal, as well as where and how the animals were housed (crowded or isolated, noisy or quiet), also influenced how susceptible the animals were to the diseases.

Is there a relationship between stress and cancer?

There have been several studies on the subject of stress and personality behaviors and their influence on cancer. Some researchers feel that major events, such as personal losses or separations, are factors in the development of cancer. Others claim there is a cancer personality, which relates loss to repressed emotions and makes such persons more cancer prone. On the other side, some scientists feel that studies relating cancer to stress are not valid, that the studies on stress and psychosocial behaviors have shown a relationship to other conditions—such as ulcers, heart disease, and mental illness—but have not yet proven a link between stress and cancer. There are currently many other studies being performed to assess the relationship.

What do animal studies show on the subject of stress and cancer?

The results of the animal studies are very confusing. They show that a variety of tumors are affected, both positively and negatively, by a variety of stressful stimulations. For instance, restraint and electric shock inhibit growth of a particular mammary tumor in rats, whereas forced swimming and handling cause the same tumor to grow more rapidly. No one knows why, and there are as yet no confirmed general principles that could predict even the direction of the effect on different tumor types of different stimulations. Although the available data provide a compelling case for psychobiological effects of cancer in animals, the complexity of both the immune system and the neuroendocrine system means that much more work is needed before definite conclusions can be drawn in this exciting area of research.

Is there such a thing as a "cancer personality"?

Some studies on cancer patients' personalities indicate that people may be more prone to cancer if they are depressed and despairing, have suffered loss or traumatic separations, or are hopeless and despondent. A study of thirty-three leukemic children found that over 90 percent had experienced a traumatic emotional loss or move within 2 years before the leukemia was diagnosed. A study of medical students found that the group with major tumors lacked closeness to one or both parents during childhood.

Other researchers have found no differences in personality between people who develop cancer and those who don't. For example, a Finnish study of depressed patients found no difference in cancer rates between them and the general population.

Since most of the studies that show personality differences have been done on patients after they already have cancer, it is difficult to determine whether there is a cancer personality or a personality brought on by cancer—whether the disease causes the emotions or vice versa. More recent studies are focusing on persons before they become ill and should help clarify the ambiguous evidence.

If there is possibly a cancer personality, are there personality traits associated with other diseases as well?

Over the years, scientists have linked certain personality traits with various diseases. The seventeenth-century physician Thomas Willis described diabetes as being caused by "an ill manner of living, sadness, long grief." Sadness and long grief have continued to be viewed as components of the diabetic personality, as have passivity, depression, stress, and apathy.

The arthritic personality has been defined as typified by depression, repression, stress, and anxiety. Emotional traits such as anxiety and guilt have been claimed to bring on skin disorders. Migraine sufferers are still thought by many to be perfectionists and success-oriented individuals.

Some studies have found that Type A individuals, who are by nature tense, short-tempered, aggressive, and always in a hurry, are two to three times more likely to have heart attacks. Type A individuals are also more prone to peptic ulcers. And young women who are high achievers and usually self-demanding are most likely to have irritable bowel syndrome.

Women with menstrual disorders can frequently be characterized as young, dependent, introverted, and immature, with a dominant mother. Infertility has been linked to young women who have been made to feel ambivalent toward reproduction and motherhood by a dominating or rejecting mother. People with high susceptibility to infectious disease appear to have had dominating or rejecting parents who led them to feel dependent and helpless.

In 1701, Dr. D. Gendron of London wrote that women with serious depression and high anxiety were prone to cancer. In 1759, Richard Guy, a surgeon, noted that malignancies occur in women with "hysteric and nervous complaints" and are peculiar to "the dull, heavy, phlegmatic, and melancholic," especially those who have met with "disasters in life and occasion much trouble and grief." In 1846, W. H. Walshe, commenting on his English patients, noted that "moral emotions (mental misery, sudden reverses of fortune, habitual gloominess) produce 'defective innervation' . . . which in turn causes the formation of carcinoma."

The question of personalities and diseases has always been controversial. Sir William Osler, the father of modern medicine, noted that "The care of tuberculosis depends more on what the patient has in his head than what he has in his chest." On the other hand, some scientists feel that the emotional difficulties are the effects rather than the causes of disease—especially since so many diseases claim the same personality traits. There is need for research that differentiates and clarifies the relationships between the emotional responses to life events and the physiological processes that occur in the development of disease.

How is imagery used in cancer therapy?

Carl Simonton and Stephanie Matthews Simonton pioneered work with patients in lifestyle counseling; this technique uses relaxation and a form of positive thinking called *imagery*. Patients are taught how to visualize strong disease-fighting white cells eating up weak, confused cancer cells. This visualization technique is combined with activities and treatments designed to teach people to live in more healthy ways. Patients are encouraged to identify and get rid of pent-up negative emotions and unhealthy behavior that might have weakened their immune systems, and to be more demanding, more expressive, and more openly angry where appropriate. The Simontons believe there is a cancer-prone personality, defined as someone who has a poor self-image, bottles up resentments, has trouble forming long-term relationships, and might have lost a serious love object or life role 6 to 18 months before diagnosis.

Does stress affect genital herpes?

Researchers at the Langley Porter Psychiatric Institute in California have found that common stresses of daily living can be a factor in altering immunity in patients with genital herpes. Both stressful experience and negative mood appear to be linked to changes in a measure of immunity: the number of helper and suppressor T cells. This is the first study to document a link among three factors: stress, immunological changes, and disease. Earlier studies linked stress and immune changes or stress and disease but never all three factors.

Can injury or trauma affect the immune system?

Doctors have long known that severely injured patients often develop pneumonia or other infections as they lie in the hospital recovering from their accidents. Dr. Eufronio Maderazo, of Hartford Hospital in Connecticut, has shown that trauma itself damages the body's infection-fighting system, leaving the victim open to invaders. Maderazo found that trauma slows the ability of white blood cells to fight germs. The patients he studied—all of whom were young, otherwise healthy victims of blows that broke bones or ruptured internal organs without causing open wounds—developed infections, most within a week of their injuries. Maderazo found that the patients were developing infections even though their white blood counts remained high. When he measured the different functions of white blood cells, he found that those in the trauma patients, within hours of their accidents, were not moving quickly enough through the walls of the blood vessels to surround and digest the invading germs. He also found that the killing ability of the white cells decreased after injury. The white cells moved more slowly in the more severely injured patients, whose infections were also worse.

Stress Experiments and What They Have Shown

- In the mid-1960s scientists at the University of Pennsylvania found that rats given electrical shocks they could not escape became passive. In the late 1970s these researchers found that when rats were injected with tumor-causing cells and subjected to inescapable shock, a high percentage of them developed tumors. The rats able to escape to another part of the cage tended to reject the tumor cells. Several researchers have shown that stress directly interfered with the body's defenses by crippling lymphocytes and other white blood cells.

- Researchers at Carleton University in Canada did repeated experiments injecting laboratory mice with cancer cells. Some of them were given electric shock to test their reactions to stress, some of them were tied down, and others were allowed to escape. The mice who were stressed and tied down developed tumors faster and died sooner. The other stressed mice who were allowed to escape did no more poorly than the unstressed mice. Researchers feel that it is how one copes with stress, rather than stress itself, that determines whether one gets sick and how serious the illness is.

- Scientists at Beth Israel Hospital in Boston and at other major centers have shown that meditation can reverse some of the dangerous aspects of the stress response. Heart and breathing rates can be lowered, cells use less oxygen, blood lactate is lessened—all signals of decreases in central nervous system activity.

- Research at the University of Rochester has shown in animals that it may be possible to learn to control the immune response through conditioned response. This is reminiscent of Pavlov's experiments, which conditioned dogs to salivate at the sound of a bell they had learned to associate with food. Mice with autoimmune disease were given saccharin along with an immunosuppressant drug. Later they were given only the saccharin, without the immunosuppressant drug. Their immune systems continued to be suppressed—having been fooled into acting as if they were responding to the drug even though it wasn't given. The saccharin-conditioned animals had less-active diseases and lower death rates.

- Researchers at the Ontario Cancer Institute in Toronto have conducted conditioning experiments with mice by giving them skin grafts from genetically different mice. These grafts produced strong immune system responses to reject the transplants. The mice then had surgical casts put around their abdomens. Following several operations, the researchers put only the surgical casts on the mice, without performing the skin grafts. Blood tests showed that the level of lymphocyte precursors (cells that mature into lymphocytes) in the mice getting just casts were three times as high as normal—the same level as when the grafting operations were performed.

- Cell biologists in Boston have found that the corticosteroids tend to depress the body's immune system, shrinking the thymus gland. If the stress is not prolonged, the thymus gland seems to recover.

- Steven Schliefer and his colleagues at Mt. Sinai Hospital in New York City studied the immune systems of hospitalized patients who were acutely ill but not on medication. They found that the patients had lower T- and B-cell response to stimulation and fewer circulating lymphocytes than did a matched group of controls. The patients under study also had higher levels of cortisol in their blood than patients in the control group (cortisol can suppress immune response). People who are very depressed have also been reported to be more susceptible to viral infections such as herpes.

- A study of healthy students conducted by scientists at Beth Israel Hospital in Boston found that those students who reported high levels of psychological symptoms in response to events that were stressful had only one-third the level of natural killer (NK) cells as did students who had little psychological reaction to the same stressful events.
- Research conducted at the Pacific Northwest Research Foundation in Seattle found that mice in a protected environment grew fewer tumors than those in the conventional small cages. This same group of researchers has shown that stressed mice experience a dramatic increase in the blood levels of corticosteroids, the adrenal hormones that can impair immune response; a decline in white blood cells, which can fight disease; and a loss of tissue from the thymus gland, which controls immune response.
- Timing of stress was another variable noted in the Seattle experiments. Stress given to mice after a tumor virus was injected made the cancer grow faster. If given before, it inhibited the growth. If the stress went on for a long time, the tumors remained smaller and the mice lived as long as did the unstressed mice. The reasons why this occurs are under further investigation.

Carcinogens, Mutagens, and Radiation

What is a carcinogen?

A carcinogen is any agent that is known to cause cancer. Many substances we take into our bodies fall into this category: tobacco smoke, radiation, sunlight, drugs, excess fats, chemicals, hormones, industrial pollutants, and polluted water. Many of our lifestyle choices—such as the amount of stress in our lives, how much alcohol we drink, and the viral diseases to which we are exposed—are believed to have carcinogenic effects on our bodies.

What is a mutagen?

A mutagen is a chemical or physical agent that causes a change in form, quality, or some other characteristic. In genetics, it is a permanent, transmissible change, usually in a single gene, that damages DNA, the genetic material.

If a substance can cause structural changes in the genetic material of a cell, it is considered to be a mutagen. Because mutations in genetic material are thought to play an important role in the development of cancer, substances that are mutagenic may be carcinogens. In animal experiments, between 80 and 85 percent of mutagens prove to be carcinogens as well.

What are the natural carcinogens and mutagens in our food?
Plants in nature create poisonous chemicals in large amounts, apparently to defend themselves against the millions of insects, bacteria, and fungi. Bruce Ames, chairman of the Department of Biochemistry at the University of California, Berkeley, estimates that our daily intake of nature's pesticides is probably 10,000

A total of some 15,000 food additives appear in foodstuffs available on American supermarket shelves, as a result of new food-processing methods.

---

times higher than our daily dietary intake of man-made pesticides. The toxic chemicals created by plants in nature are manufactured by the plants to ward off insects and fungi. The plants also contain anticarcinogens. Most researchers feel that much remains to be discovered about the extent to which naturally occurring chemicals appear in food, whether they are actually cancer producing, the significance of eating mutagens, and the means of counteracting any harmful effects.

How serious a threat to good health are natural mutagens and carcinogens?
Researchers have found that natural carcinogens may be as threatening to good health as man-made ones. Bruce Ames now feels that concentrating exclusively on pollution and man-made chemicals, while ignoring the vast amounts of natural mutagens and carcinogens, may be the wrong path to take.

Is there a health risk to everything we eat?
No human diet can be entirely free of carcinogens or mutagens. Dietary practices are being carefully scrutinized by scientists to determine what foods and cooking methods are most beneficial to health. Since comparisons of data from different countries show wide differences in rates and types of disease, it is hoped that many may be avoidable with a change in dietary habits. There is increasing evidence that large numbers of potent carcinogens are generated by natural processes. Mutagens are present in substantial quantities

in fruits and vegetables. Carcinogens are formed in cooking as a result of reactions involving proteins or fats.

What are some examples of naturally occurring mutagens and carcinogens in the human diet?

The variety of toxic chemicals manufactured in nature is tremendous. Although organic chemists have been analyzing them for over 100 years, toxicological studies have been completed for only a very small percentage. Dr. Bruce Ames of the University of California at Berkeley recently listed the following sixteen examples of the natural mutagens, teratogens, and carcinogens in the human diet:

1. Safrole, estragole, methyleugenol, and piperine. (Oil of sassafras, used in natural sarsaparilla root beer, contains safrole. Black pepper contains both safrole and piperine.)
2. Hydrazines are present in edible mushrooms.
3. Psoralen derivatives are present in celery, parsnips, figs, and parsley, particularly if the plants are diseased.
4. Solanine and chaconine, potato glycoalkaloids, can reach lethal levels when potatoes are diseased, bruised, or exposed to light.
5. Quercetin and similar flavonoids are present in buckwheat, tea leaves, and hops.
6. Quinones and their phenol precursors are found in rhubarb and mold toxins, caffeine components, benzene, and cigarette smoke.
7. Theobromine is present in cocoa and tea.
8. Pyrrolizidine alkaloids are present in herbs and herbal teas and occasionally in honey.
9. Vicine and convicine are present in the broad fava bean.
10. Allyl isothiocyanate is used as a flavor ingredient in oil of mustard and horseradish.
11. Gossypol is a major toxin in cottonseed. (This substance is being tested as a male contraceptive in China, as it is inexpensive and causes sterility during use. Plant breeders have developed "glandless cotton," a new strain with low levels of gossypol, but seeds from this strain are susceptible to attack by a fungus that produces the potent carcinogen aflatoxin.)
12. Sterculic acid and malvalic acid are toxic fatty acids present in cottonseed oil, kapok, etc., and may be ingested from

consumption of fish, poultry, eggs, and milk from animals fed with cottonseed.

13. Leguminous plants such as lupine, which animals feed on in winter, are known to cause an abnormality called "crooked calf." In one rural California family, a baby boy, a litter of puppies, and goat kids all had "crooked" bone birth defects. During pregnancy the mother and the dog had both been drinking milk from the family goats. It had first been thought that the defects were the result of spraying of 2,4 D, but later study showed that they were caused by the goat milk—and that the goats had been foraging on lupine.

14. Sesquiterpene lactons, which cause the bitter taste in many plants, are a major toxin in the white sap of *Lactuca virosa* (poison lettuce), which has been used as a folk remedy. Plant breeders are transferring genes from this species to commercial lettuce to increase insect resistance.

15. Phorbol esters, used as folk remedies or herb teas, may be the cause of nasopharyngeal cancer in China and esophageal cancer in Curaçao.

16. Canavanine, a highly toxic arginine analog, is found in alfalfa sprouts. It appears to be the active agent in causing the severe lupus erythematosus-like syndrome that occurs when monkeys are fed alfalfa sprouts.

How does sunlight affect the immune system?

Ultraviolet rays may suppress the body's immune system, according to studies at the Frederick Cancer Research Institute in Maryland. Normally the body's T lymphocytes destroy cancerous cells before they cause any problem. However, ultraviolet light causes special suppressor cells to be produced, and these cells prevent the T cells from doing their job.

How does the moon affect health?

Ulcer research has shown that patients with bleeding ulcers are more likely to suffer a crisis during the period of the full moon. Similarly, epileptics are more likely to have a convulsive attack, and diabetics have more problems. There is a higher incidence of strokes and attacks of angina pectoris. Dr. Ralph W. Morris, professor of pharmacology at the University of Illinois, reported that in a study of eighty-eight patients, 64 percent of the angina attacks occurred between the full and the last-quarter phase. Studies performed on rodents by the same group of researchers found that morphine given at full moon made rodents feel less pain without losing consciousness nearly 70 percent of the time, compared with about 50 percent during new-moon periods. During full-moon periods, people seem to have higher metabolism rates and increased tensions and anxieties. Hormones are more active, heart rate is at its peak, blood pressure is up, and hair growth seems more active. The strongest change in behavior seems to occur in people who are high-strung and nervous. They become more assertive and aggressive.

> • In North Carolina, over 250 medical students were measured for hostility. Those who scored highest had five times the number of heart problems.

Can blood transfusions suppress the immune system?
Yes. Both human and animal studies have shown that blood transfusions can suppress activity in the immune system, reducing the body's defenses against infection and other foreign substances. In the 1970s, studies indicated that kidney transplant patients who were given blood transfusions before surgery were less likely to reject the organ. Several recent studies from the University of Vermont, Mt. Sinai Medical Center in New York City, and the University of Rochester Medical Center suggest that cancer patients who receive blood transfusions at the time their tumors are surgically removed have a significantly greater chance of early recurrence and death from the disease than other patients. Researchers, who note that the findings are preliminary, feel that blood transfusions may adversely affect the body's natural defenses and its response to tumor growth. It is not known whether it is the blood transfusions or other factors that are responsible for the differences among surgery patients treated for different forms of cancer.

Does radiation affect the immune system?
Yes. Even at low doses, radiation has a lethal effect on lymphocytes and immune system cells in general. The most radiation-sensitive lymphocytes appear to be suppressor cells. Microscopic examination of tissues that have been irradiated reveals chromosomes that are broken or rearranged and repaired.

Is radiation good or bad?
Unnecessary or excessive exposure to radiation is dangerous. The

evidence that radiation is a carcinogen is overwhelming, and radiation overexposure does result in malignant tumors. However, the judicious use of radiation, both for diagnosis and treatment, is beneficial, and not using it can expose a person to greater risks than the radiation itself.

The following are known facts about radiation:

- Radiation affects the ability of the immune system to perform because it has lethal effects, even at low doses, on lymphocytes and immune stem cells in general.
- Chromosomes are broken and rearranged in tissues that have been exposed to radiation.
- Persons with Down's syndrome (mongolism), Fanconi's anemia (a rare hereditary disorder), Bloom's syndrome (dwarfism with defects in skin pigmentation), and ataxia-telangiectasia (a progressive failure of muscular coordination) are very sensitive to radiation and show a high incidence of tumors after exposure. All of these disorders are characterized by a large number of breaks in the chromosomes that are either unrepaired or misrepaired.
- Age at time of exposure is a major factor. For instance, the risk of radiation-induced breast cancer is highest in those exposed between the ages of 10 and 19. It decreases steadily until age 50, when it starts rising again. Studies on leukemia induction show that fetal exposure, even at low doses, results in higher risks. Risks are still high but not as great when exposure occurs in the first years of life.
- In general, there is a consistent increase in cases of tumors for each increase in radiation dose.
- Single doses of 400 rads produce no increase in cases of breast cancer in rats and, in fact, may decrease the rate—and may decrease the rate of other nonmalignant tumors.
- Lowering the rate at which a given dose is delivered has a sparing effect. This is probably due to cellular repair processes.
- Although in cell cultures, cell survival increases when the doses are fractionated (divided into smaller amounts and given at intervals), some researchers have found that those cells that survive at low doses and low dose rates are more likely to become cancerous.
- Many chemotherapeutic drugs act as negatively as would another dose of radiation in areas that have already been irradi-

ated. Some act to increase the radiation effects in addition to the effects of the drugs.

The sites most sensitive to tumors as a result of radiation are lung, marrow, and colon. All of these also have a high spontaneous incidence of cancer. Skin, prostate, and cervix, which also have a high spontaneous incidence of cancer, are not as likely to develop tumors from radiation exposure.

Is radon a naturally occurring substance?
Yes, it is. Dirt and rock surrounding the foundations of thousands of homes emit radon, according to toxicologists. Radon is a naturally occurring radioactive product that may cause lung cancer in nonsmokers.

Do chemicals alter the immune system?
Studies have found that some chemicals alter the immune systems of mice. In patients, both stimulation and suppression of the immune system can be triggered by drugs and chemicals. What is not known is the long-term impact of the alteration. Many researchers are studying specific cause-and-effect relationships in mice between their exposures to varying levels of chemicals and the impact on their immune systems. Determining the dose-response relationship of toxic materials and recommending safe exposure levels is at the heart of a new discipline called immunotoxicology—the scientific marriage of immunology and toxicology.

Are all chemicals carcinogenic?
No, they are not. When the National Cancer Institute tested 150 industrial compounds and pesticides, selected because of suspicions as to their possible carcinogenicity, less than 10 percent of them were found to be carcinogenic.

What toxic chemicals are being released into the air by manufacturers?
To what extent hazardous material is released into the air from factories and other plants is unknown. There are presently few regulations on most pollutants. One reason for the lack of clear standards is the controversy among scientists over what levels are safe for the population. A congressional survey of eighty-six large chemical companies reported that chemicals such as chloroform, chlorine, benzine, and carbon tetrachloride were being emitted by sixty-seven of the companies.

Are there dangerous toxins in our homes?

A 5-year study by the Environmental Protection Agency reported that toxic chemicals in the home—chemicals as common as paint and cleaning solvents—are three times more likely to cause cancer than airborne pollutants, even in areas located next to chemical plants. Americans appear to be exposed to surprisingly high levels of toxic chemicals in their homes through cooking, drinking water, skin absorption, and breathing. The nationwide drive to save energy—sealing windows and doors and insulating walls and roofs—has trapped many of the pollutants inside. Researchers found little difference in the levels of such contaminants as benzene and tetrachloroethylene when they compared indoor levels of pollution in homes close to chemical plants to those of homes far from heavy industry. The total number of chemicals found in common household products amounts to more than 50,000 different substances.

Coffee, Alcohol, and Smoking

Does coffee cause mutagens?

Laboratory studies have shown that compounds contained in coffee catalyze the formation of carcinogenic nitrosamines from nitrite under acid conditions similar to those in the stomach. Studies have also shown that a class of compounds that includes caffeine cause mutations in bacteria.

Does too much alcohol in the diet affect the immune system?

There is evidence that excessive alcohol consumption depresses the inflammatory response of the body's immune system in both men and women. Some researchers feel that the fact that there is a much lower overall cancer rate among Mormons and Seventh-Day Adventists (who abstain from alcohol for religious reasons), compared with the rest of the population, is further evidence.

Is the immune system disrupted by cigarette smoking?

A group of researchers from the Massachusetts General Hospital, Harvard Medical School and Ortho Pharmaceuticals, Inc., have found strong evidence that smoking seriously disrupts the body's immune system. The team's work shows that smokers, especially those who smoke heavily, have abnormal ratios of T cells in their blood. They gathered samples from heavy smokers, moderate smokers, light smokers, and nonsmokers. The significant changes in T-cell ratios were seen only in heavy smokers—those who had 50 pack-year histories of smoking. A 50 pack-year history includes someone who has smoked one pack of cigarettes a day for 50 years or two packs a day for 25 years or three packs a day for 17 years.

People in the study group who stopped smoking were divided up according to their smoking habits. Blood tests were taken before they stopped, 3 weeks after they stopped, and again 6 weeks after smoking ended. This research showed that the abnormal condition can be reversed by stopping smoking. Blood tests indicated that when heavy smokers stopped smoking, their immune systems returned to normal within weeks.

Is smoking related to lung cancer?

All four major types of lung cancer are related to cigarette smoking in both men and women. Smokers are two times more likely to develop all cancers than nonsmokers and about ten times more likely to get lung cancer. Eighty-five to 90 percent of all lung cancers are caused by cigarette smoking. There have been eight major studies that have measured deaths among smokers and nonsmokers followed for many years from England, the United States, Japan, Canada, and Sweden. These studies represent more than 17 million person-years of observation and over 330,000 deaths. They all strongly implicate smoking as the chief cause of lung cancer. Epidemiologists have also shown that the most important cause of lung cancer is cigarette smoking and that urban factors, such as air pollution, probably contribute to less than 5 percent of lung cancers in the United States.

Is the immune system endangered by exposure to suntan-parlor tanning?

Yes. Dr. Peter Hersey of the University of Newcastle Medical School in Australia found that the immune system's ratio of helper cells to suppressor cells was depressed after suntan-parlor exposure. Suntan parlors are usually advertised as "safe" because they emit ultraviolet A radiation (called UVA), which is supposed to be less damaging than ultraviolet B (called UVB), which the sun emits. However, many of the UVA booths also give off UVB rays.

In Dr. Hersey's study, volunteers had tanned for 30-minute daily sessions for 14 days in suntan solariums with supposedly safe ultraviolet light. Not only was the helper-suppressor ratio depressed, but the depression continued for 2 weeks after the suntan-parlor exposure.

Does smoking have an effect on vitamin C levels in the body?
It has been shown that smokers have a much lower level of vitamin C in their bodies than nonsmokers. Dr. Anders Kallner of Stockholm suggests that the toxic compounds in cigarettes lower the body's reserves of vitamin C. Using a process known as isotope labeling, he was able to measure exactly how much vitamin C was lost or retained by the body, and how much was required to maintain the body's reserves at a sufficient level. He concluded that the Russian recommended daily allowance (RDA) of about 100 milligrams was much nearer the true requirement than the U.S. RDA of 60 milligrams. For smokers, however, at least 140 milligrams a day is indicated.

Does marijuana affect the immune system?
It is known that chronic or long-term use of marijuana weakens the immune response and that users have less resistance to infections and other diseases.

Studies in Hawaii show that different ethnic groups are susceptible to different cancer incidences.

Hawaiians have the highest stomach cancer rates but the lowest colon cancer rates.

Filipino women have the highest thyroid cancer rates but the lowest breast cancer rates.

Migrants to Hawaii show dramatic shifts in cancer rates compared with those in their country of origin and with their children born in Hawaii.

Studies are investigating lifestyle differences such as smoking, drinking, sunbathing, and diet to determine which of these factors had an influence.

Anesthesia and Pain

Do studies show a correlation between the immune response and the nutritional status of patients undergoing surgery?
A June 1983 report in *Surgery* points up a correlation between the immune response, the nutritional status of the patient, and the incidence of wound complications in patients undergoing vas-

cular operations. Seventy-nine patients were closely followed, and the researchers were able to statistically analyze a number of medical measurements to try to find a way of reducing problems following surgery. Many of the patients had been in nursing homes and all were aged 70 or older, had required repetitive vascular surgical procedures within a short period of time, and had already had wound problems. It was found that among the patients with delayed healing or wound infection the serum albumin level was below 3 grams. Those with serum albumin levels higher than 3 grams were found to be more likely to have uncomplicated wound healing. Also, the development of wound complications was much more likely in patients whose transferrin levels were lower than 150 milligrams. Since serum albumin and transferrin are two major, easily measured secretory proteins that serve to transport metals, ions, drugs, hormones, and metabolites, the value of keeping a close check on these levels before surgery is performed seems to be indicated. It is interesting to note that four patients who were in serious condition and required emergency aortic reconstruction and who were excluded from the final study because they received immediate and aggressive forced supplemental nutrition and feedings all had successful outcomes to their surgery, pointing to the importance of nutrition in strengthening the immune response.

Does anesthesia affect the immune system?
Anesthetics involve all cells to some extent, so the cells involved in the immune system are affected. Anesthesia also stimulates the stress response and this effect, interwoven with surgery, produces more specific and more complex changes in the immune system. Exposure to anesthesia and surgery results in depression of the immune system, but the results appear to be short-lived and relatively minor. However, there are longer-term immunosuppressive effects of steroids released as part of the stress response to anesthesia and surgery. It is theorized that the primary cause of depressed resistance to infection after surgery may well be the stress reaction to surgery rather than the drugs used during the surgical procedures.

Is the way anesthesia works a clue to how it affects the immune system?
Researchers are still trying to solve the mystery of how anesthesia performs its functions. They know that acetylcholine is a com-

mon neurotransmitter that carries out a variety of messenger duties in the body, such as stimulating lymphocytes to prepare to fight foreign substances. Anesthesia desensitizes acetylcholine receptors, so it is possible that this action may in some way weaken or depress the immune system following anesthesia.

Does pain affect the immune system?
It has been found that pain, particularly after surgery, may suppress the immune system and delay recovery. Restoring immune functions as soon as possible is related to early movement and general recovery from an operation. Vitamin A has been found to counteract the postoperative decrease of immune response.

Fat, Vitamin and Mineral Deficiencies

Is there a connection between malnutrition and the immune system?
There has been considerable research with children who live in areas of the world where malnutrition is a problem. The results of this research provide an indication of the relationship of diet to the immune system.

Ranjit Chandra (University of Newfoundland) has done research in India. He notes that the thymus is extremely sensitive to malnutrition. Children and adults who have both protein and calorie malnutrition also have deficiencies in their immune systems. When infections occur, they lead to more severe malnutrition and a greatly suppressed immune function. Chandra emphasizes the importance of nutrients such as iron, zinc, and vitamin A, which may influence immunity and which may be deficient in children with malnutrition.

Chandra further notes that babies who were small for their date of birth also had immunological deficiencies that are corrected only very slowly by nutritional rehabilitation. In these infants, low T-cell numbers present after birth persisted for periods of time ranging from several months up to 5 years.

E. Richard Stiehm, of the University of California at Los Angeles, studied malnourished hospitalized children in Los Angeles and found that the numbers of lymphocytes and T cells in their blood were low and that the low number of T cells was correlated with their susceptibility to infection.

Robert Good, formerly of Memorial Sloan-Kettering Cancer Center in New York City, found that restriction of zinc in the diets of both animals and humans lowered function of the thymus, development and function of T cells, and activity of helper cells. Replacing the zinc in the diets of animals and humans corrected the functioning of the thymus and T cells and restored the numbers and functions of lymphoid cells.

Does the amount of calories or fat in the diet have any effect on the immune system?

According to a report in *Nutrition Reviews* (April 1982), studies performed on a strain of mice with short life spans showed that restricting the calories and fat in the diets of mice of this strain doubled their life spans and retarded the development of all diseases associated with aging, including deficiencies in the immune system. Feeding such mice a diet high in fat speeded up the development of the deficiencies in their immune systems as well as the development of the diseases of aging.

Experiments performed by Dr. Ludwik Gross of the Veterans Administration Medical Center in Bronx, New York, showed that tumors were produced in 100 percent of rats allowed to eat their fill (about five or six pellets of rat food a day) and given a dose of X rays. When the same dose of X rays was given to rats whose diet was limited to two pellets of food a day, only nine out of twenty-nine females and one out of fifteen males developed tumors. The weight of the rats on the reduced diet fell by about one-half, but they remained healthy and outlived their counterparts who died of cancer. The research also found that the restricted diet reduced the occurrence of benign tumors. However, there was no evidence that restricting food slowed the growth of tumors that had already formed in the rats.

Why is a fatty diet considered a health hazard?

Fats vastly increase the secretion of digestive chemicals—namely bile acids and steroids—into the intestines. Apparently this chemical flood damages the walls of some intestinal cells and causes the immune system to be less effective.

Does diet play any role in causing cancer?

The relationship between diet and cancer has not yet been precisely defined, but research increasingly points to the role of diet in causing cancer. The National Cancer Institute's latest figures (1984) show that about 80 percent of cancer cases can be linked to lifestyle and environmental factors in the following proportions:

35% to diets, especially those low in fiber and high in fat
30% to smoking
5% to viruses
4% to occupational exposures
3% to excess sunlight
3% to alcohol
2% to environmental pollution
1% to food additives

What kinds of cancers are associated with a high-fat diet?

Cancers of the breast, colon, and prostate have been associated with high fat diets. The United States National Research Council has judged that the evidence for fat as a cause of human cancer, particularly of the colon and the breast, is sufficient to recommend a reduction in dietary intake of both saturated and unsaturated fats.

During World War II in England and Wales, there was a marked decrease in deaths due to cancers of the breast and colon. Consumption of cereal products, fruit, and vegetables increased 25 percent during wartime, while fat consumption decreased 18 percent. After the war, when dietary fat and fiber content went back to prewar levels, deaths due to these two cancers increased.

High levels of dietary fat seem to enhance the development of both spontaneous and chemically induced breast cancers in mice. The highest tumor production occurred when the fat was fed both before and after the exposure to the cancer-inducing chemical, lending support to the theory that dietary fat acts as a cancer promoter.

Countries with the highest fat consumption also have the highest breast cancer mortality. If you compare the countries with the highest fat intake with the countries that have only half that fat intake, you find breast cancer deaths twice as high in the high-fat countries as in the low-fat countries.

A study by National Cancer Institute (NCI) scientists in eastern Nebraska found an increased risk for colon cancer in patients with a high-fat diet, particularly when the fat was obtained from meat, dairy products, and sweets.

NCI scientists are studying the possible association of diet and lifestyle with decreased risk for certain cancers. Maps of cancer mortality in the United States, based on data collected between

1950 and 1969, showed that death rates from colon, rectal, and breast cancers were about 50 percent lower in the southern states than in the northeastern and north-central regions. Despite the large number of northerners who retired to Florida, this area seemed to retain the low rates of the South, even among older people. The researchers are investigating whether the risk for colorectal cancer can be rapidly reduced by environmental and dietary influences.

How does a high-fat diet promote cancer of the breast?
According to Clifford Welsch, Ph.D., a tumor biologist at Michigan State University, the high-fat diet promotes the secretion of hormones that stimulate the development of hormone-responsive breast tissue—both normal and cancerous. It is Dr. Welsch's opinion that a high-fat diet increases the susceptibility of the breast tissue to hormone stimulation.

Does the way foods are prepared have an influence on cancer?
Because consumption of foods high in fat has been strongly linked to a number of cancers, cooking methods that minimize the use of fats and oils are recommended. These include steaming, boiling, stewing, slow cooking in a crock pot, and microwave cooking. Steaming, baking, and sautéing vegetables also helps preserve vitamins and other nutrients.

Charcoal broiling and grilling meat can produce potentially harmful substances from the fat and protein in meat. Melted fat dripped onto hot coals is converted to carcinogenic benzo[a]pyrene, which then contaminates the meat as it is carried up by smoke. The breaking down of protein by heat also forms mutagenic compounds.

Despite the presence of mutagens in broiled foods, epidemiologic studies have failed to show a link between the consumption of these foods and gastric cancer. Americans eat relatively large quantities of broiled foods, yet the incidence of gastric cancer has dropped dramatically in the last few decades.

Does severe constipation seem to be a factor in the development of cancer?
Researchers at the University of California at San Francisco found that women with severe constipation (two or fewer bowel movements a week) were five times more likely to show signs of possible abnormal cell growth in breast fluids than were women with normal bowel functions. It is possible that estro-

gen secreted by the liver is reabsorbed more readily with sluggish digestion.

Do vitamins have an effect on the immune system?

The subject of vitamins and their interaction with the immune system is a very complex one. Some studies have already demonstrated the importance of vitamins, and much additional research is currently underway. According to an article in *Nutrition Reviews* (April 1982), based on a major international conference of nutrition scientists, research has yielded the following information:

- Deficiency of a substance in vitamin B_6 (pyridoxine) may produce serious problems in the workings of T cells.
- Deficiency of vitamin B_{12} can lead to defects in several parts of the immune system, including neutrophils, T cells, and monocytes.
- Deficiency of folic acid (part of the B-vitamin group) can lead to less resistance to infection, lowered production of antibodies, and defects in the responses of the thymus and the lymphocytes.
- Deficiency of vitamin C weakens the ability of the body to generate an immune response.
- Vitamin A deficiency profoundly influences T-cell immune function, and increased intakes of vitamin A are claimed to stimulate immunity.
- Vitamin E stimulates the functions which increase the ability to fight infections.
- Some amino acids have significant influences on the functions of the immune system (amino acids form the chief structure of proteins).
- Some unsaturated fatty acids suppress the immune system; and the higher the unsaturation, the greater the suppression of the immune system.
- Many minerals—such as iron, zinc, magnesium, selenium, and iodine—affect immunity.

Do vitamin needs increase with age?

While good nutrition cannot guarantee perfect health or reverse the aging process, it can help forestall the diseases of aging. Determining vitamin needs at any age is far from simple. Even when meals are well balanced, older people may face other problems—such as malabsorption, which can decrease vitamin availability, particularly of fat-soluble vitamins A, D, E, and K as well as folic acid and vitamin B_{12}. Alcohol interferes with the absorption of a number of nutrients, and has emerged as a major cause of thiamine and folic-acid deficiency in older people. Multiple drugs over long periods of time and the use of therapeutic agents including laxatives, anticonvulsants, and diuretics can also hamper vitamin utilization.

> Repeated studies show that pickled vegetables and dried, salted fish appear to have a direct relationship to stomach cancer, particularly in men. An increased intake of vitamin C, shown in case-control studies among Japanese in Hawaii, helps reduce the incidence of stomach cancer.

What is the relationship of zinc to the immune function?
There is little doubt that zinc is intimately involved in immune function. The importance of zinc for the normal growth of plants was first recognized over 100 years ago—and it has since been proven that zinc is required for the activity of over seventy enzymes involved in cell division.

Voluminous research shows that zinc is an absolute requirement for proper lymphocyte balance. Though studies of the direct in vitro effect of zinc upon purified T and B lymphocytes are in their infancy, the dietary research seems to indicate that there is a definite correlation between T lymphocytes and zinc. It has been shown that depressed zinc supply can have an adverse effect on recovery after surgery. In one study, with patients who had head and neck surgery, there was a pronounced drop in zinc levels, which persisted for at least 30 days in one-third of the patients, accompanied by impaired wound healing and depressed cellular immunity. Both healing ability and cellular immunity improved with the addition of zinc supplements.

Can zinc shortage in the diet weaken body immunity?
It has been known for 20 years that zinc is an important nutrient, but its role in immunity has become clearer since research has accelerated on AIDS (*a*cquired *i*mmmune *d*eficiency *s*yndrome). Abnormalities caused by zinc deficiency are very similar to those caused by AIDS. Both AIDS and zinc-deficient diets affect the workings of the thymus gland, which is responsible for the proper

growth of T cells. However, the proper amount of zinc must be determined, as it has also been shown than an overabundance of zinc acts to depress the immune system.

What are nitrosamines?

Nitrosamines are potent carcinogens that can form in the stomach. When nitrates—a family of chemicals found in some water supplies and in some green vegetables, cured meats, and cheeses—combine with bacteria in the mouth, different compounds known as nitrites may form. The nitrites, in turn, combine with components of some foods, drugs, and other substances to form carcinogenic nitrosamines. Vitamin C appears to serve as a natural defense against nitrosamines by preventing their formation in the body. Studies in several countries have shown that eating fresh fruits and vegetables containing vitamin C helps reduce the risk of stomach cancer.

chapter 3

Strengthening Immunity the Natural Way

What we all really want to know is "How do I make myself more immune to all the threatening diseases there are in this world?" Looking at the research, it is clear that, although the path is by no means a straight and simple one, there are a variety of guiding signposts. The most exciting news is that, given an understanding of how the immune system works, there are specific ways in which we can help ourselves to bolster our immune systems.

It is now known that in the very first days of life the nursing baby's immune system receives special help from the colostrum in the mother's breast milk. Designed to confer several months of early immunity, the colostrum transfers antibodies directly from mother to baby, to bolster the baby's immune system until it begins to produce its own antibodies.

Even ancient healers and medicine men were aware of the link between emotions and disease, and scientists are now able to document how emotions—especially responses to stress—affect the immune system. Learning new ways of handling stress—such as biofeedback, yoga, hypnosis, and relaxation techniques—can make a difference.

There is little question that emotions and health are closely related. It has been known for many years that negative emotions and experiences can have an adverse effect on health and can complicate medical treatment. Not as well known is the connection between positive attitudes and the possible enhancement of the body's healing system. It is likely that numerous emotional and physical factors, many of them yet to be delineated, influence health and disease, probably in different ways for different individuals.

In addition, throughout life, proper nutrients, including vitamins and minerals, clearly have an effect on keeping the immune system in tip-top shape. More scientific evidence is being uncovered on how increasing the intake of specific vitamins and trace minerals can play a role in enhancing immunity.

Many simple, natural methods of strengthening the immune system are being rediscovered, scientifically investigated, and explored. It is possible that in the future we may learn to treat disease by fine-tuning brain chemicals. Meanwhile, we owe it to ourselves to investigate the many natural means of stimulating the immune system and then to determine how we can fit them into our own lifestyles.

Acquiring Immunity:
Disease, Vaccination, Breastfeeding

What is active immunity?

There are two types of active immunity. The first results from actually having had a specific disease. The body reacts by producing enough antibodies to overcome the infecting viruses or bacteria. The second kind of active immunity is produced deliberately by injecting vaccine made from dead, weakened, or live bacteria or viruses or from toxins and toxoids (toxins that have been made less irritating). Immunization also enables the body to produce antibodies rapidly and in large amounts when the immunizing substance is injected again within a limited period of time. This is known as the booster or recall reaction.

What is colostrum, and what are its effects on the nursing baby?

Colostrum is the yellowish fluid that is produced by the breasts shortly after the birth of a baby. It contains up to 20 percent protein, predominant among which are immunoglobulins, representing the antibodies found in the mother's blood. Colostrum contains more minerals and less fat and carbohydrate than the mother's milk, which is not secreted until several days after birth. Through the colostrum, the mother is able to transfer her antibodies and other protective substances that destroy viruses, bacteria, and other microorganisms, giving the newborn extra protection until his or her own system is able to take over.

In a study of mothers with pre-term pregnancies (36 weeks or less), marked differences in the immunologic characteristics of their milk were found in comparing it with the milk of mothers whose babies were full term. IgA concentration in the pre-term milk was found to increase substantially between 8 and 12 weeks; also, the milk of the pre-term mothers had much lower leukocyte counts, which gradually increased up to 12 weeks. The conclusion of the scientists was that the immunologic composition of human milk depends not only on the period of lactation but also on the length of the pregnancy.

It has been found that breastfed babies are less likely to have runny noses, eczema, and other allergic symptoms than bottle-fed babies. A substance called the bifidus factor, contained in the mother's milk, promotes the growth of harmless bifid bacteria in the intestinal tracts of breastfed babies.

Immunity and the Mind

Does the brain exert control over the immune system?
John Liebeskind, a psychologist at the University of California, Los Angeles, is fascinated by the possibility that the brain can exert control over the immune system, meaning that our health might be determined by our training. Some biologists go so far as to claim that psychological therapy that teaches people how to feel in control of their lives might in some measure prevent disease and act as a valuable supplement to conventional medical care. Detailing the direct relationship of the brain to the immune system is still in the future, since it has not yet been proved that an individual emotion sparks a direct bodily response—although the signals are clear. It is known that electrochemical activity in the brain causes the hypothalamus to trigger the release of adrenocorticotropin (ACTH) from the pituitary gland. This hormone travels in the bloodstream, reacting in the kidneys and ultimately prompting the adrenal glands to release hormones like cortisol and epinephrine, which can affect almost every organ.

How is information transmitted within the brain?
In the brain are more than 100 billion nerve cells. Almost none of the nerve cells in the brain quite touch each other, yet connections exist. Electrical impulses move from nerve cell to nerve

cell and are carried across the gaps between them by special chemicals called neurotransmitters. Each of the 100-plus billion nerve cells in the brain is connected to an average of 1000 other neurons, making the brain an electrochemical computer—more complex than any computer ever built.

Is there evidence that the brain can be trained to exercise control over the immune system?

It has been shown in experiments that the two hemispheres of the brain influence the immune system in different ways. In research experiments conducted at the University of Alabama Medical School, mice were exposed for 3 hours at a time to the odor of camphor. The camphor itself had no detectable effect on the immune system. In the experiments, some mice were given injections of a synthetic chemical known to enhance the activity of natural killer cells. The exposures to the odor and the injections were repeated nine times. In the tenth session the mice were exposed only to the odor of the camphor; they received no injections. Nevertheless, every mouse showed a large increase in natural killer cell activity.

In a follow-up experiment, further refinements were made in the research. Some animals were exposed to the odor of camphor and given injections in each of the sessions, then, in the tenth session, they were not exposed to the odor and were given injections of salt water. When the two groups were compared, it was found that those given only the exposure to camphor in the tenth session had three times the amount of natural killer cell activity as the animals in the other group. The links between the brain and the immune system are just beginning to be explored, though they have been pondered from the earliest recorded time.

Does the brain control the immune system, or does the immune system control the brain?

There seems to be evidence that the brain and the immune system are in continuous communication. Scientists at George Washington University have found thymosin—a hormone produced by the thymus, the gland responsible for the specialization of some lymphocytes as T cells—in the brain. One theory is that thymosin travels from the body to the hypothalamus to the pituitary; that there it may influence the release of the chemicals that trigger the release of cortisol into the blood. The theory continues that cortisol is not merely an immunosuppressant but, rather, a regulatory hormone.

What are endorphins?
Endorphins are chemicals in the body. They come in at least three different types and many subtypes. All have druglike properties, similar to heroin or morphine. Endorphins were first discovered in the mid-1970s, and research is just beginning to reveal the ways in which they work. By acting to slow down the transmission of information, endorphins play a role in controlling pain. Ongoing research into the role of endorphins is widening to include studies of mental illness, memory and learning, arthritis, obesity, compulsive running, the menstrual cycle, dealing with stress, and the functioning of the immune system.

What effect do endorphins have on the immune system?
Some experiments suggest that endorphins influence the immune system by increasing the disease-fighting responses of T cells. Others show that the endorphins that are released under stress suppress the immune function, decreasing the effectiveness of the natural killer cells. Some researchers believe that endorphins may act to release or modify the release of other hormones that directly suppress the activity of the immune system. The field of research on endorphins is young, and many new developments are needed before we understand the exact relationship of endorphins to the immune system.

Is there any evidence that being left-handed has an effect on the immune system?
A Harvard neurologist, Norman Geschwind, feels that during the fetal development of left-handers, the left side of the brain may be slowed down by higher levels of testosterone, the male sex hormone. Testosterone is known to alter the development of the immune system, both before and after birth. Very strongly left-handed people are more likely to suffer from allergies, ulcerative colitis, and other autoimmune diseases than are right-handed people or those who use their right hands for some tasks. However, Dr. Geschwind feels that left-handers may be less susceptible to some infections and cancer.

Immunity and Stress

Can a person learn to control his or her own immune system?
This question is being widely researched. Tests in animals show that it may be possible to control the immune system through conditioned response. Some researchers feel that there will even-

tually be a way to teach people to exert control over their own immune systems, but whether or not the release of hormones can be controlled by a person and used to cast off disease is a topic that requires extensive research. By testing people's reactions to stress, it may be possible to identify markers that can predict who is more likely to develop certain diseases. It may then be possible, for instance, to train people at risk to suppress their own destructive immune reactions or to treat allergy-sensitive people whose immune systems react to innocent substances.

One interesting study by psychologist Robert Ader of the University of Rochester School of Medicine and his colleague, immunologist Nicholas Cohen, dealt with a strain of mice that develop a type of lupus. They injected the mice with an immunosuppressive drug and coupled it with a drink of saccharin solution. At random, saline injections were substituted for the drug. The conditioned mice developed symptoms much more slowly than did untreated controls. More significantly, their mortality rate was no higher than that of animals that were given the drug each time. The saccharin solution apparently signaled the mice's bodies to suppress the immune response even in the absence of the drug.

What research is being done to determine how attitudes affect cancer?

Numerous studies are under way—and some have been completed—to delve into this controversial subject. One study recently published by a team led by Dr. Barrie Cassileth at the University of Pennsylvania Cancer Center in Philadelphia, developed questionnaires that were administered to 204 patients with very advanced cancer and to 155 patients who had been treated either for breast cancer or for melanoma, both of which are cancers that often recur. Cancer victims were questioned about lifestyles and feelings concerning their health, their jobs, their degree of hopelessness or helplessness. This particular study drew the conclusion that the more cheerful patients showed no greater capability than the depressed ones for fighting their cancers, and that the pessimists appeared to be at no greater risk of death or recurrence than the optimists. The medical profession continues to debate the study. Some emphasis has been placed on the damage done by placing the further burden of having to accept responsibility for the spread of disease upon a patient who is already suffering from the disease process.

Other studies—many already completed, some still under way—however, have come to the opposite conclusion. Most physicians instinctively feel that a strong will to live helps a patient's chances in combating serious illness. Proving this point in a scientific manner, however, is a more difficult matter. The truth is that at present it is not known to what extent psychobiologic factors contribute to the induction and progression of, or recovery from, disease. Only after much more information is available will we be able to separate fact from folklore.

Is there a link between illness and emotions?

The idea of a link between emotions and disease has been with us since the ancient healers and medicine men. However, it is only within the past few years that scientists have been able to document how emotions, acting through the brain, can affect hormone levels, the immune response, and the functioning of the nervous system. These new studies show that many illnesses, from the lowly cold to heart disease, have a mind/body link. The research is part of a new field of investigation called psychoneuroimmunology (PNI), which studies how it is possible for the mind to influence the immune system. Its parent field, neuroimmunomodulation, enfolds a whole range of studies based on viewing the brain as a computer that is involved in all the other reactions of the body. The research recognizes the fact that the endocrine system, the nervous system, and the immune system are part of a totality.

What is PNI?

PNI, a term that is probably as unfamiliar to most doctors as it is to most laypeople, stands for psychoneuroimmunology. Research into the area shows that emotional states, behavioral patterns, and mental attitudes are central issues in health and disease. The pathways in the body include neurological connections linking the body's glands and organs with the brain through the blood, by means of hormonal secretions triggered by thought patterns and emotions. In a pioneering study carried out over 20 years ago, Dr. David Kissen, a Scottish researcher, examined more than 1000 industrial workers suffering from respiratory complaints. Before diagnosing them, he gave them a psychological test designed to delineate personality patterns. He came up with some significant results, discovering that those who were later found to have cancer showed a striking inability to express their emotions. PNI researchers are currently investigating a variety of mind/body techniques that can alter the mental attitude and emotional states from negative to positive and therefore encourage good immune functions and protection from illness.

What is Norman Cousins' theory of the relationship between mental attitude and physical health?

Norman Cousins, author of *Anatomy of an Illness* and former editor of the *Saturday Review,* has written of his own personal experiences with serious illness and how positive emotions and the patient/physician partnership cured him of spinal arthritis. He called attention to research showing that laughter can enhance respiration and, in some cases, stimulate the endocrine system.

Do emotions such as anxiety, apathy, and depression have an effect on the immune system?

It appears that these emotions may have a significant effect on immune system factors such as the natural killer cells that fight cancer. Research studies also show that there are links between the emotions and such diseases as flu, colds, and genital herpes.

Is there any evidence that positive attitudes can reverse cancer malignancies?

There is insufficient evidence so far to indicate that positive attitudes alone can reverse cases of advanced malignancies. However, some remissions and unexpected recoveries do occur, and medical science continues, while treating the physical side of the disease, to investigate the possibilities of how the mind influences health. Even where positive attitudes and good mental outlook cannot influence the physical outcome, scientists and physicians agree, they can and do have an effect on the quality of life.

Does the support of family and friends make a difference in stress situations?

Studies indicate that it does. Population studies in California have investigated how lifestyle behaviors might influence health. Focusing on health practices such as exercise, cigarette smoking, alcohol use, and patterns of sleeping and eating, the researchers found that people with good health practices had much lower death rates than those with poor health practices. The study also recorded information on the social networks of the participants: immediate family, close friends and relatives, and affiliations with organizations such as churches and clubs. The people with good social networks had lower death rates than the people who did not have good social networks. Those with weak social networks and poor health practices were found to be five times as likely to die as those with good health practices and strong social networks.

Does the way an individual reacts to stress have any bearing on the immune system?

What is perceived as stress differs from one person to another. What is stressful to one may actually be stimulating to another. The student whose grade for the entire semester depends upon a certain test score feels a different stress than the student for whom the same exam is not crucial. The student who feels well prepared for a test is not likely to feel as highly stressed by the test as the student who does not feel well prepared, regardless of how much each has studied. The way a person perceives his ability to cope with a specific demand influences how stressed he feels about it. Many researchers believe that how a person *responds* to the events in his life, rather than the events themselves, influences susceptibility to disease. Coping well with a high-stress life may actually be protective.

Can researchers categorize stress?

Some researchers are suggesting that stressful events be categorized according to how a person feels about them: good or bad, controllable or uncontrollable, intense or mild. Others feel that the duration of the stress plays a major role; they break stress into four categories: emotions, moods, emotional traits, and emotional disorders, with each type lasting for a longer period than the preceding one. For instance, sadness would be an emotion, but depression would be an emotional disorder. Only traits and disorders, these researchers feel, have long-term health consequences.

Can we learn to make stress a positive rather than a negative force?

Yes. Stress is part of life. It can be an immensely productive part if used properly. We must learn to channel stress, to take pleasure in successes, and to recognize the early-warning signals of stress and the ways it can be avoided. We can use stress to make us stronger and healthier. According to Susan Seliger, author of *Stop Killing Yourself: Make Stress Work for You,* researchers have found that the chemicals released in the response to stress vary slightly depending on whether you feel happy or sad, as though you can cope or you can't cope. She feels that "successfully rising to a challenge and feeling that glow of confidence and a sense of control over one's destiny seem to go a long way toward counteracting the ill effects of stress. It may even help cure disease." An insurance company study of over 1000 men in top executive positions found their death rate to be 37 percent lower than that of other men of the same age. A phone company study of over 250 executives found that people who were able to handle stress, no matter how much pressure they were under, all had the same attitude: they felt in control in their jobs, with a sense of purpose, and viewed change as a challenge, not a threat.

Are there studies that show specifically measurable effects of what stress does to the immune system?

One series of studies conducted by Janice Kiecolt-Glaser and Ronald Glaser, a husband-and-wife team at Ohio State University School of Medicine, has found that the stress surrounding academic examinations has specifically measurable effects on the immune systems of students. They found a decline in the aspects of immunity, including the ability to produce interferon, that are involved in fighting off infection and disease.

Are there any specific skills a person can learn to control stress?

Charles Stroebel, an expert in stress physiology and the author of *QR, the Quieting Reflex,* developed QR by studying the immediate response of the human body to stress. QR is intended to counteract the first 6 seconds of the body's response to a stressful situation (the fight-or-flight reflex) by substituting opposite body reactions, thus preventing the reflex from occurring. He suggests that as soon as you get the clue that something is causing you to feel stressed you:

- smile inwardly and with your eyes and mouth, to counter facial tension.
- give yourself this suggestion: "alert, amused mind, calm body."
- take an easy, deep abdominal breath.
- exhale, letting your jaw, tongue, and shoulders go limp. Feel the wave of heaviness and warmth flowing through your body to your toes.

• go back to your normal activity.
• keep practicing so that it becomes an automatic response to stressful situations without your even thinking about it.

Are there ways to alter some of the personality traits that seem to be linked to disease?
People can certainly learn to deal with some of the emotional responses that make up their personality types. The challenge is to work at becoming a happier person, because happy people tend to be healthy. To maintain a positive, self-confident view of life, try to:

• exercise at least three times a week. Walk, swim, ride a bicycle, play a sport—but do something.
• take stock of your past achievements and enjoy them.
• learn how to relax. Go into a quiet room and blot out distractions for 10 or 15 minutes. Or do relaxation or meditation exercises daily.
• get rid of your negative emotions. Talk out your feelings or confront people as soon as they make you angry. Learn not to overreact emotionally.
• plan leisure time so you can recharge your batteries.
• stop doing things you don't enjoy.
• draw up a set of goals to help you achieve what you want in the way of a career, personal growth, or relationships with others.
• decide the things you have to do and the things you want to do and feel good about succeeding in them.
• learn to cope with stressful events. Take action instead of standing by doing nothing to help yourself.
• work at having good relationships with friends or family members on whom you can count for support.

Is there any evidence that grief affects the immune system?
The intense grief that people endure at the loss of a loved one may have measurable biological effects on hormone and brain functions, and consequently on the immune system in susceptible persons. Researchers at the University of California at San Diego, in a study dealing with people seeking psychiatric help, found that unresolved grief lingered for 10 years or more and was associated with complaints of depression and a number of physical

symptoms. In this study the majority of deceased relatives were either fathers or mothers.

A report issued by the National Academy of Sciences documents the observation that there is an increase in serious illness and early death for bereaved persons, especially men. Scientists believe that some biological predisposition might determine which persons find bereavement particularly difficult. Those with a history of depression, or whose families include members with histories of depression, appear to be most vulnerable.

Two other separate but related studies now under way, conducted by the National Institute of Alcohol Abuse and Alcoholism and the National Institute of Mental Health, are attempting to pinpoint the neuroendocrine abnormalities that may govern one person's reaction to the loss of a loved one, or push another into uncontrollable compulsive gambling. The scientists will examine blood samples for biological evidence suggesting depression and high levels of stress.

Biofeedback, Yoga, Acupuncture, Hypnosis, Acupressure, Color, Light

Can the sympathetic nervous system be controlled through biofeedback?

Several scientists have demonstrated that the sympathetic nervous system can indeed be controlled through biofeedback. Biofeedback can help a person to understand that the mind and body work together. People can already be taught to affect the temperature of their hands through visualizing warm or cold. Biofeedback has helped demonstrate that stress situations can cause hand temperature to drop, showing the close relationship between the body and the mind. Several experts have shown that chronic stress can result in increased production of steroids from the adrenal system and that autogenic training can reduce the level of circulating cortisol. Relaxation techniques, self-hypnosis, and biofeedback are becoming more and more widely used. However, the idea of enhancing the immune system through relaxation or the possibility that the immune system can respond to pictures in the mind are concepts that require further scientific research.

How is biofeedback being used in treating asthma?

In the treatment of bronchial asthma, biofeedback is used to give specific information about actual resistance to airflow to the lungs and to help teach general relaxation and measure its effect. Ongoing research focuses on developing biofeedback equipment as well as on the body functions, responses, and techniques.

How is yoga used to enhance health?

Yoga, which has been practiced for over 5000 years, is called a science for the whole body, including the mind. Persons who practice it feel it works to achieve total health because it is a science of how to stay healthy. There are several different types of yoga:

Hatha yoga (*ha* = sun, *tha* = moon) is a program of exercises designed to keep the body healthy through flexibility and the balancing of the body's natural heating and cooling mechanism. Flexibility is intended to increase the body's general resistance to disease by keeping the lymph circulating properly, with the belief that good circulation strengthens the body's immune system. Alternate-nostril breathing is used to aid digestion and the proper functioning of the nervous system. Breathing through the left nostril is said to cool the body, while breathing only through the right will tend to raise the heat level.

Raja yoga (yoga of kings) works for the mind instead of the body. It tries to make the mind flexible and also less receptive to stress or depression, through meditation and the deliberate attainment of mental control.

Bhaktai yoga works to develop one's love of self and fellow humans.

Karma yoga deals with a person's attitude toward work and play, attempting to reconcile them until there is no such thing as an unpleasant task.

Can acupuncture have an effect on immune defenses?

The answer to that question is not yet known. There is little hard scientific evidence that acupuncture works—although the method has been in use for 5000 years in China. Some recent studies done on pain indicate that natural brain opiates are perhaps stimulated through acupuncture. Experiments done on both cats and humans have verified the fact that a neurochemical is involved, and it appears that the pituitary gland and midbrain release a chemical during and following acupuncture.

Bruce Pomerantz at the University of Toronto has researched acupuncture by recording electrical impulses. His work has shown that the pain-relieving effects of acupuncture may be caused by stimulating the brain to release endorphins. Chinese doctors have demonstrated that a painkilling chemical is present in the brain, and other research teams have verified that such chemicals are the endorphins. More research will be necessary to develop the theory further. The mere fact that little scientific evidence is available that acupuncture techniques activate deep sensory nerves indicates how little we truly know about the functioning of the body.

Can hypnosis and acupuncture prevent pain?

Neither hypnosis nor acupuncture can produce anesthesia, but both can produce an absence of the ability to feel pain. For this to happen, there must be some traffic between the connecting cells of the nervous system. For instance, if fluid from the brain and spinal cord is transferred from an animal on which acupuncture is being performed, to another animal, the other animal receives some painkilling effect. Researchers feel that the painkilling effect is produced by the release of endorphins. The painkilling effect of hypnosis, researchers believe, is caused by a blockage of the nerve fibers. Hypnosis can modify allergic skin responses and symptoms of allergic asthma and hay fever. Researchers feel that the immune response can be modified by hypnosis even though the mechanism is probably very different from that of anesthetic drugs.

How is acupressure used to stimulate the immune system?

Acupressure is a harmless self-help technique of fingertip stimulation in which small pressure points located near the surface of the skin are briskly massaged. It is an ancient Chinese method, related to acupuncture. As in acupuncture, the bioenergy in the body is thought to have a definite, predictable route through the body, flowing along a pathway in a fixed pattern, with important terminals where the bioenergy changes direction along the pathway. The specific points (acupoints) are believed to be directly responsible for the manner in which the bioenergy reaches the organs. Pressure points, because of their broad-acting, pressure-responsive nature, can be used to stimulate the immune system and for temporary relief of numerous symptoms.

Acupressure Points

Exact pressure points vary from person to person. To find yours, probe deeply around the area until you find the most sensitive spot, which will announce itself with a distinct twinge.

Technique is easy to learn. Apply pressure with the tip of the index finger—not the flat pad of the finger. Don't just rub and move skin, but apply solid pressure in a circular motion to the spot. Long fingernails get in the way. Usually fingertip pressure is sufficient, but if you feel more pressure is needed, use the flat end of a felt marker, your thumb or your knuckle.

In order to accurately locate pressure points, remember that the width of one hand refers to the distance across the four middle knuckles of the fingers. The width of the thumb refers to the distance across the widest part of the thumb.

To complete the treatment, fifteen or twenty seconds worth of pressure is recommended. It must be done twice, once on the right side of the body and once on the left. It doesn't make any difference which side you do first, but it should be followed with identical pressure on the opposite side.

1 **COLD SYMPTOMS** This point is located at the top of the wrist in the small hollow at the apex of lines drawn from the thumbnail and the index finger. Can be located by placing hands on top of each other, linking thumbs. Index finger of top hand can probe and find the spot. Repeat on opposite wrist.

2 **HEADACHE** On the top of the hand, trace up from the middle finger to a spot about two finger widths above the prominent crease of the upper wrist. Repeat on opposite wrist. (Massage of the lower earlobes is also suggested.)

3 **TENNIS ELBOW** Easiest way to find this point is to bend the arm tightly and place your finger at the extreme end of the crease. Keeping your finger on the spot, straighten the arm and stimulate the point on your relaxed arm. Repeat on opposite arm.

4 SORE THROAT Stimulate the spot directly between the thumbnail and knuckle on the side away from the fingers. Repeat on other hand.

5 TEMPER CONTROL, ANXIETY ATTACKS This one is on a line with the small finger, on the crease of the inner wrist. Repeat on opposite wrist.

6 MOTION SICKNESS You'll find this spot in line with the middle finger, on the inner wrist, two thumbs above the prominent crease of the wrist. Repeat on other wrist.

7 COUGH OR LARYNGITIS Inside of arm at the elbow crease, in the hollow. Usually located toward the outer side of the arm. Don't forget to repeat on other arm.

8 BACKACHE, especially low back pain. This one is above the heel, in the area of the outer ankle, in the depression behind the curved end of the shin bone knob. Repeat on other leg.

9 INDIGESTION OR HUNGER PANGS On the inside of the ankle, measure the width of one hand above the shin bone knob. The pressure point is at this height, toward the front of the leg, just behind the bone. Repeat on other ankle.

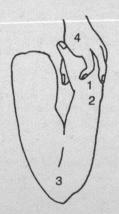

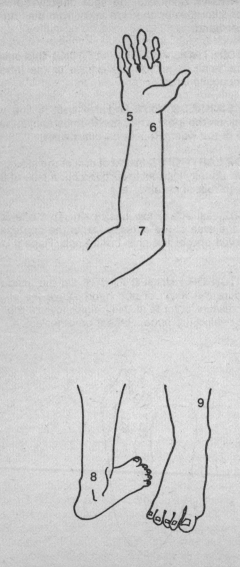

Is it possible that color has an effect on body chemistry?

A number of studies over the years have shown that the body is sensitive, through the eye, to color. Each of millions of colors is a distinct wavelength of light that strikes color-sensitive cones on the back of the eye in a unique way. These cells send nerve signals to the brain. It is possible that this process may trigger the release of hormones or neurotransmitters, which in turn influence body activities such as heart rate and breathing. Baths of light emitting a high concentration of blue wavelengths are now used in many hospitals to cure infants of neonatal jaundice. The light penetrates the skin and breaks down the chemical bilirubin, which causes the condition. Of course, there is much debate within the medical profession regarding the legitimacy of color as a health tool, but it is another area to be considered in the entire picture of how the brain affects the body systems.

Does light affect the immune system?

It is not yet known what effect light has on the immune system. There is, however, research being done on a syndrome know as SAD—seasonal *affective* *disorder*. Psychiatrists are finding that gloomy winter moods can be quickly and completely dispelled with light. Researchers have studied the role of melatonin, a hormone that is produced only at night, to determine if blocking its synthesis would lift the depression. These studies have failed to support the theory, indicating that something in addition to melatonin was at work. Scientists are now looking at the neurotransmitter serotonin and how it may be related to SAD. Serotonin is found in all parts of the brain and has been linked to sleep cycles, carbohydrate craving, appetite satiety, feelings of contentment, and pain relief, among other things.

The average Chinese herb shop carries a selection of about 2000 different items—a variety of herbs and other native plants used for medicinal purposes in different regions. These natural compounds actually form the basis for many of our present-day medicines. Chamomile tea is known to contain substances that have a tranquilizing effect—and offer another route to the solution of problems of sleeplessness and anxiety. Spices have been used for thousands of years in food preservation. Many spices are antioxidants; they preserve food in the same way as synthetics such as BHT or BHA. Cloves, oregano, sage, rosemary, and vanilla are all classified as antioxidants.

Dietary Fiber and Fat

What is the relationship of dietary fiber to cancer?
Dietary fiber is a component of food that is largely indigestible
and provides bulk in the diet. It is found in vegetables, fruits,
and whole-grain cereals and includes indigestible carbohydrates
and carbohydratelike components of food such as cellulose lig-
nin, hemicelluloses, pentosans, gums, and pectins. Fiber consists
of plant walls and nonnutritive residues, including all substances
resistant to animal digestive enzymes.

Most studies of the possibly protective effect of fiber against
colon cancer have found that intestinal diseases such as appendicitis, diverticulosis, and colonic polyps as well as colon cancer
occur less frequently in populations that consume large amounts
of fiber in the diet. If there is a fiber component that protects
against colorectal cancer, it may work by hastening the travel
time of fecal matter through the bowel (so that food carcinogens
are in contact with the bowel mucosa for less time), by increasing
the bulk of the stool (thus diluting the concentration of carcinogens), or by changing the species of the bacteria in the bowel (to
a form that may destroy cancer-causing metabolites or is less
likely to form fecal mutagens).

Does it make any difference what kind of fiber you eat?
It seems to. In animal studies, it has been reported that the protective effect of fiber depends on the kind of fiber. One set of
researchers compared the effects of two different kinds of fiber
on chemically induced colon cancers in male rats. Both fiber types
reduced the cases of small tumors of the colon, compared with a
control diet without the fibers. The fibers differed with respect to
their effects on the concentration of fecal bile acids and total bile
acids.

Both the Mormons and the Seventh-Day Adventists have a low
incidence of colon cancer and a diet high in fiber, including fiber
from fruits and vegetables as well as fiber from grains. The National Cancer Institute recommends that the average American
should increase fiber intake from the present level of 10 to 20

grams a day to between 25 and 35 grams a day. You can do that by adding three more fibrous foods each day. For example, a bowl of whole-fiber cereal with a sliced banana or berries adds two fibrous foods. Try to eat whole-grain breads and cereals and fruit and/or vegetables at each meal.

Can fiber protect against the effects of fat in the diet?

International studies of human populations indicate that fiber may offer protection from the adverse effects of fat. Which type of fiber and how fiber affords its protection are not yet fully known. In a study comparing Finnish and Danish population groups, which have similar dietary intakes of fat, colon cancer incidence was much lower among the rural Finns, whose diet contains large amounts of high-fiber, unrefined rye bread than among the Danes in Copenhagen, who have a low-fiber diet.

In animal studies, fiber has provided either partial or complete protection against the effect of fat on the incidence of chemically induced colon cancer in rats. The rats were fed one of five semi-synthetic diets containing various amounts of fat and fiber. The incidence and number of tumors per animal increased in all fat-fed groups. Adding fiber to diets provided partial protection against polyunsaturated fat and complete protection against saturated fats.

What are the most common sources of fat in the American diet?

The most common sources, in order, are:

    ground meat
    hot dogs and luncheon meats
    full-fat dairy products
    cookies and other pastries
    ice cream and frozen desserts
    salty snacks such as potato chips and nuts
    fried chicken and fried fish
    gravy and meat sauces

If your diet is high in one or more of these categories, you should choose a leaner version of the food, eat less of it, or replace the food with another that serves the same dietary purpose but provides substantially less fat. Most Americans would benefit greatly by cutting their fat intake in half—from 42 percent of total calories to between 20 and 30 percent of total calories.

Are there any studies of the effect of a low-fat diet on breast cancer?

A major study, the Women's Health Trial, is examining the effects of a low-fat diet on breast cancer. High-risk women—those who have two first-degree relatives with breast cancer, or have one first-degree relative with breast cancer and two or more biopsies for benign breast disease, or were 30 or older at the time of their first pregnancy—will be studied to see if reducing fat in the diet from the present average 40 percent of calories to closer to 20 percent will reduce the incidence of cancer among these women. This study will take ten years to complete.

Vitamins

Which vitamins are most important in enhancing the immune system?

The vitamins that play the greatest role in strengthening the immune system are beta carotene, B_1, B_2, B_5 (pantothenic acid), B_6, and C. Zinc, a mineral, is also important.

What is the Recommended Dietary Allowance (RDA) of vitamins and minerals?

Commonly known as the RDA, the Recommended Dietary Allowance is the official standard for nutrient requirements recommended by the Food and Nutrition Board of the National Academy of Sciences/National Research Council. It is a broad guideline for the average daily amounts of nutrients that people should consume, based on an intake of about 2000 calories a day. It provides nutrient guidelines in amounts sufficient to prevent definite deficiency conditions such as scurvy, pellagra, or beriberi—but not necessarily to promote optimum health. The RDA is used in setting standards for package labeling and for large-scale menu planning for schools, hospitals, the military, and prisons. It does not take into account variations in individual needs or in individual eating patterns. Women who are chronic dieters, pregnant and nursing women, users of birth control pills, smokers, heavy drinkers, and the elderly are at increased risk for deficiencies. The Department of Agriculture, in preparing suggested diets below 1600 calories daily, found it impossible to assure RDA levels of all essential nutrients. Since about half of all American women consume fewer than 1500 calories a day, it is almost a certainty that many are significantly deficient in many essential nutrients.

Why do people need vitamin supplements?

We all know that if we eat a well-balanced diet there is no need for additional vitamins. A well-balanced diet is described as at least four servings of grain and cereal products; four or more servings of a variety of fruits and vegetables; two servings of dairy products; and two of meat, fish, or poultry. The only problem is that most people regularly just don't eat as well as they should. If you are on a strict low-calorie diet or are a picky eater, supplementing your diet with a multivitamin pill probably makes good nutritional sense.

Are megadoses of vitamins a good substitute for those who don't get enough vitamins from food?

The best way to obtain your daily vitamin ration is to eat a wide variety of foods. For those who may feel they are not getting enough vitamins, a multivitamin supplement, as close to the appropriate RDAs as possible, is a safe hedge against deficiency. Most experts agree that you'll be safe taking a supplement containing up to twice the RDAs. What should be avoided, unless under a doctor's prescription, is megadosing. Megadosing is defined as taking ten times the RDA for water-soluble vitamins and five times the RDA for fat-soluble vitamins. Taken in megadose quantities, some vitamins can be toxic and cause unpleasant or dangerous side effects.

What's the difference between fat-soluble and water-soluble vitamins?

Fat-soluble vitamins are stored in the body's fat—so they do not necessarily have to be consumed every day. Water-soluble vitamins must be consumed daily in adequate amounts to meet the daily need, since they are continually being washed out of the body with urine and sweat.

Which vitamins are fat-soluble?

A, D, E, and K are the fat-soluble vitamins. Because they are stored in the body, there is a danger of overdosing with fat-soluble vitamins, so caution must be used.

What are the water-soluble vitamins?

The eight B-complex vitamins and vitamin C are all water-soluble. Large percentages of these vitamins are lost during food processing, preparation, and storage. Often the water in which vegetables are cooked contains more vitamins (which are discarded) than are finally available when the food reaches the table.

How does vitamin A affect the body?

Vitamin A is a powerful immune-system stimulant. It has been shown to increase the size of the thymus gland, one of the important components of the immune system. Vitamin A can prevent the decrease in the size of the thymus that normally occurs after injuries. It has been used to decrease the development of cancer in animals exposed to cancer-causing chemicals. A derivative of vitamin A is used in treating acne. Vitamin A works better when it is taken with a chelated-zinc supplement.

Is beta carotene the same as vitamin A?

Beta carotene is a common source of vitamin A and is found in leafy green and yellow vegetables, certain fruits, liver, and dairy products. The beta carotene found in leafy green and yellow vegetables is converted to vitamin A in the digestive tract. It is uncertain whether beta carotene's association with reduced cancer risk is due only to its conversion to vitamin A or whether beta carotene has some protective effect of its own. Many studies have reported a relationship between low risk for cancer and high consumption of foods containing beta carotene. Epidemiologic studies in Norway and the United States showed that smokers who consumed low amounts of vitamin A had a somewhat higher risk of lung cancer than those who consumed adequate amounts.

What are the most popular sources of beta carotene?
Carrots account for the major source of beta carotene in the diets of Americans. In Japan, yellow and green vegetables provide the major source of this important fat-soluble vitamin. In West Africa, red palm oil is the most important source of beta carotene. Large daily doses of natural beta carotene appear to be harmless and the body seems to convert to vitamin A only what it requires, so there is no fear of developing vitamin A toxicity from eating an overabundance of foods containing beta carotene.

Are retinoids also vitamin A?
Retinoids are derivatives and chemical cousins of vitamin A. Several animal studies have shown that vitamin A and the retinoids can prevent and reverse chemically induced lung tumors. However, natural retinoids are known to have toxic effects in animals, particularly at high doses. Researchers are now trying to develop synthetic retinoids that are as effective as natural retinoids in preventing cancer growth, less toxic, and more specific to different cancer sites. A new synthetic retinoid that appears to meet these criteria is 4-HPR (4-hydroxyphenyl retinamide). It has been shown to prevent the development of breast cancer in the rat and bladder cancer in the mouse. In early testing in England it has been shown to have very low toxicity compared with more standard retinoids such as vitamin A or the retinoic acids. Based on this evidence, the National Cancer Institute is supporting trials to test its effectiveness against bladder and breast cancer in humans.

What diseases can be caused by vitamin A deficiency?
New studies in Third World countries have found that dietary deficiencies of vitamin A are a major cause of blindness and are responsible for significant increases in measles, diarrhea, and other potentially deadly diseases in children in Africa, Asia, and Latin America.

On the island of Sumatra, in Indonesia, death rates among poor children who received vitamin A therapy were one-third lower than among children who did not receive the supplements. Night blindness, which causes children to stumble about at twilight, and xerophthalmia, a permanent blindness, result from inadequate vitamin A. Children of the poor and landless are most susceptible, since they have the least access to green leafy vegetables, fruits, milk, eggs, liver, and fish, which provide the vitamin.

Scientists do not know exactly how vitamin A deficiency promotes the potentially deadly diseases. Some feel it might be because the immune system is suppressed. Researchers found that children with night blindness died at a higher rate than other children. The more severe the vitamin A deficiency, the higher the death rate, especially from respiratory diseases and diarrhea. Giving vitamin A supplements reduced the death rate by 35 percent.

Can vitamin A prevent cancer?

A growing number of laboratory and human studies indicate that there may be some connection between vitamin A and cancer prevention. About twenty studies undertaken in various parts of the world suggest that eating foods containing vitamin A or beta carotene might reduce the risk of developing cancer by some 30 to 50 percent. For instance, several controlled studies show lower vegetable consumption or lower estimates of vitamin A intake among patients with cancer than among controls. Three studies—one of 8278 Norwegian men, another of 265,118 Japanese adults, and the third of 2107 American men—found a higher risk of lung cancer among those who ate food containing vitamin A.

Bjelke in Norway showed that male smokers who consumed low amounts of vitamin A had a somewhat higher risk of lung cancer than those who consumed adequate amounts of vitamin A. Carrots, milk, and eggs were the main source of vitamin A in the men studied. This 1975 study was recently updated and expanded, and its findings were confirmed at the Thirteenth International Cancer Congress. The Hirayama study in Japan involved adults who filled out a dietary questionnaire in their 1965 census. The development of cancer was documented over a 10-year period. Daily consumption of vegetables high in beta carotene was linked with a decreased risk of developing cancers of the lung, colon, stomach, prostate, and cervix. Shekelle and colleagues in the Illinois study suggest that the benefit may be related more to the dietary vitamin A precursor beta carotene than to vitamin A itself.

Does vitamin A protect against cancer?

Most studies show that it does. Graham, Mettlin, and colleagues at the Roswell Park Memorial Institute in Buffalo, New York, have conducted nine dietary studies on people who already have cancer. Overall they found an increased cancer risk in those who had the lowest levels of vitamin A intake. The authors speculated that vitamin A may have a cancer-protective effect in such organs as the lung, bladder, mouth, esophagus, larynx, breast, and uterine cervix. A study of diet and cancer of the mouth and throat showed differences in adult food intake between women with cancer and normal women without cancer from the southern United States. High consumption of fruits and vegetables seemed to have a protective effect. Some studies have found that the vitamin A effect appears to be smaller in males than in females. The National Cancer Institute's position is that the evidence thus far available suggests (though it is not definitive) that beta carotene is truly protective against cancer and that the question cannot be definitely decided until the results from the current human trials become available.

Can vitamin A or vitamin E induce an immune response to cancer?

Maurice Black, M.D., of the Institute for Breast Disease at New York Medical College, is using short-term oral doses of both vitamins A and E in women who have had one breast cancer. Participants in the research are women who do not naturally show a strong immune response to their cancers. It has been found that 50 to 60 percent of the women show an immune response when they start taking large doses of either A or E and that the response shoots up to 80 percent when both A and E are taken. It is not known whether the induced response works as well as a spontaneous response or whether there is a reduced incidence of recurrent or second primary breast cancer.

What are some of the current human trials that will give us definitive future proof of the protection of Vitamin A?

Ziegler, Mason, and coworkers in the NCI's Environmental Epidemiology Branch, in collaboration with the New Jersey Department of Health and the University of Texas School of Public Health, are conducting a study to assess the relative contributions of vitamin A and beta carotene in reducing the risk for lung cancer. The scientists are comparing vitamin A with beta carotene intake by interviewing living patients with lung cancer; close relatives and friends of people who have died of lung cancer; and normal people of comparable age, race, and sex in certain areas of New Jersey and the Gulf Coast of Texas, where lung cancer death rates are higher than in the United States as a whole.

Selikoff of Mt. Sinai Hospital in New York City is studying

the possible association of low levels of dietary vitamin A with lung cancer development and the potential use of measurements of blood levels of vitamin A to predict risk and guide surveillance of the high-risk group of asbestos workers.

Kjelsberg at the University of Minneapolis is evaluating the relationship between dietary intake of vitamin A and beta carotene, blood levels of vitamin A and beta carotene, and cancer. Dietary results collected annually on 12,000 men during a 7-year follow-up study of participants in a National Heart, Lung, and Blood Institute study are being used for the dietary analysis.

Is there any research on the use of vitamin A in preventing skin cancer?
There are several studies under way, including the following:

Gideon Luande of the Muhimbili Medical Center in Tanzania, East Africa, and Claudia Henschke of Brigham and Women's Hospitals in Boston are studying a population of albino Africans who lack the skin pigment that protects against the intense solar radiation near the equator and who often die from skin cancer before age 30. Patients will receive either beta carotene or a placebo.

Thomas Moon of the University of Arizona is studying the value of vitamin A in reducing the risk of basal-cell skin cancer in patients with actinic keratoses (lesions that occur on the sun-exposed skin of the faces or hands of elderly light-skinned persons and may be precursor lesions for basal-cell cancer). Moon is also investigating the safety and adverse effects of long-term doses of vitamin A and the vitamin A levels in the blood of persons in the study.

Bijan Safai of Memorial Sloan-Kettering Cancer Center in New York City is investigating whether beta carotene, or a combination of beta carotene and vitamins C and E, given to individuals at high risk for basal-cell skin cancer, may reduce the occurrence of new tumors. Safai is also studying the role of the immune system and heredity in basal-cell skin cancer and the influence of beta carotene and a combination of beta carotene with vitamins C and E on immunity.

What are the symptoms of excessive intake of vitamin A?
Vitamin A is known to be toxic if taken in excessive amounts.

Watch out for sparse, coarse hair; loss of hair on the eyebrows; dry, rough skin or skin rashes; cracked lips; severe headache; weakness; cessation of menstruation; and jaundice.

Arctic explorers have been known to suffer from the effects of high vitamin A intake from eating polar-bear or seal liver. Drowsiness, irritability, headache, and vomiting occurred; later, their skin peeled. One polar explorer died as the result of eating a liver that was estimated to contain about 100 million units of vitamin A.

How long have scientists been aware of the association between vitamin A and cancer protection?

A relationship between cancer and vitamin A deficiency was first suggested in the 1920s when Y. Fujimaki, a scientist, thought that a diet deficient in vitamin A might be the cause of stomach cancer in rats. Although a subsequent study found that it was precancer rather than true cancer, the link between vitamin A and cancer development was established.

In 1955, Ilse Lasnitzki of the Strangeways Research Laboratory in Cambridge, England, showed that precancerous changes in mouse prostate cells treated with a carcinogenic hydrocarbon could be inhibited by vitamin A.

More recently, Michael Sporn and his coworkers at the National Cancer Institute, in collaboration with Richard Moon and colleagues at the IIT Research Institute of Chicago, showed that feeding rats and mice a synthetic retinoid inhibited the development of carcinogen-induced bladder tumors. They also demonstrated that carcinogen-induced rat mammary tumors could be reduced to as low as one-fifth the expected incidence by feeding synthetic retinoids after exposure to carcinogens. Roswell K. Boutwell and his colleagues at the University of Wisconsin have shown that synthetic retinoids inhibit the later (promotion) stage of skin cancer development in mice. There are many more studies in the laboratory and in animals, all clearly showing that the effectiveness of a retinoid as a preventive agent for cancer varies with the particular retinoid, the cancer-producing agent (or carcinogen), the type of cancer, and the animal being studied.

Are the B vitamins interdependent on one another?

Yes—and excess intake of any one may create a greater need for the others. However, most excess B vitamins are excreted in the urine and do not pose a threat to health. Several of the B vitamins are important to carbohydrate metabolism, so the more sugars and starches in your diet, the more B vitamins you probably need.

What are the B-complex vitamins?

The B vitamins are a family of vitamins that includes B_1(thiamine), B_2(riboflavin), B_3(niacin), B_6(pyridoxine), and B_{12} (colbalamin). It is important to obtain each vitamin of the complex in the proper ratios in your diet. Most of the low-dosage B-complex supplements on the market have done this balancing for you. Megadosages should be scrutinized because overdoses of one B vitamin, without the supplementation of the others, may throw the interrelationship off balance, resulting in deficiencies of the others. B vitamins are water-soluble. Therefore, you need them every day. They can be washed out of your body by drinking a lot of coffee, tea, or alcohol or by perspiring heavily.

What is vitamin B_1?

Vitamin B_1, or thiamine, is essential to normal metabolism and nerve function. When it is absorbed by the small intestine, thiamine is circulated throughout the body to nourish the basic organs and body cells. It helps in the formation of ribose, a sugar vital to the manufacture of the nucleic acid RNA, which contains our genetic information. Thiamine is helpful if you are suffering from diarrhea or any other intestinal problem. It helps the body make the most efficient use of the nutrients it does absorb and protects against a secondary ailment. Pork, liver, oysters, whole grains, brewer's yeast, seeds, and nuts are all good sources of vitamin B_1.

What is vitamin B_2?

Vitamin B_2, or riboflavin, is a growth-promoting member of the vitamin B complex. It works with vitamin A in providing normal vision and is essential for the assimilation of iron. It helps promote proper growth of cells, tissues, and organs. If vitamin B_2 is not available, the enzymes cannot perform the necessary chemical reactions to release energy; thus, the body's entire energy cycle is interrupted or slowed. B_2 works in the red blood cells to keep them healthy.

Inadequate B_2 intake can cause disorders in blood cell formation and abnormalities in the bone marrow where the cells are synthesized. Liver, milk, whole grains, dark-green vegetables, mushrooms, and soy all supply vitamin B_2.

What is vitamin B_3?

This vitamin is also known as niacin or nicotinic acid. The body is able to manufacture B_3—although not enough to adequately supply the body's daily needs—when there are adequate supplies of B_1, B_2, and B_6. Niacin is essential to every cell in the body— and it has been found to be needed in greater-than-normal quantities by those who suffer from pellagra, mental illness, arthritis, alcoholism, high cholesterol levels, cardiovascular troubles, or chronic migraine headaches. Niacin is available in organ meats, salmon, tuna, wheat germ, brewer's yeast, green vegetables, beans, peas, prunes, and dates. Megadoses can aggravate asthma, diabetes, peptic ulcer, liver disease, and gout.

Does niacin have an effect on allergic reactions?

Niacin or nicotinic acid (but not niacinamide) can cause the release of histamine. Because niacin may release histamine, it has been suggested that caution in taking supplemental doses of niacin should be exercised by people with asthma and peptic ulcer disease. The Coronary Drug Project Group found an increase in the incidence of acute gouty arthritis in patients on high doses of niacin (3 grams per day).

What is vitamin B_6?

Vitamin B_6, also referred to as pyridoxine, assists in manufacturing DNA and RNA, the nucleic acids that contain the genetic codes for growth, repair, and multiplication of cells. A deficiency of B_6 produces an impairment in the immune response. Iron must combine with B_6 to make the hemoglobin your body requires. If B_6 is not available in adequate amounts, dietary iron will not be fully utilized. Diets rich in fat or protein, or both, contribute to the depletion of vitamin B_6 in the plasma because of the biochemical reactions involved in the breakdown and conversion of these substances. A deficiency of niacin may result when B_6 is inadequate, because niacin cannot be properly produced when levels of B_6 are low. Good sources of B_6 include the usual whole grains, beans, and fresh vegetables and meat as well as liver, avocados, and bananas.

What is vitamin B_{12}?

B_{12} is the most complex of the B vitamins—and it works in every cell of the body. It is especially vital to the cells in the bone marrow, gastrointestinal tract, and nervous system. Injections of this vitamin are given to those who suffer from pernicious anemia. B_{12} is especially important if you are a vegetarian, an alcoholic, or suffer from mental illness. B_{12} and folic acid should be taken together, since folic acid cannot be activated if B_{12} is not present. Meat, poultry, nonfat dry milk, and fermented soybean products provide B_{12}, as do liver, kidneys, eggs, milk, oysters, fish, and soy sauce.

What is pantothenic acid?

Pantothenic acid—sometimes referred to as B_5—plays a major role in the immune system. It manufactures antibodies that fight infectious compounds in the bloodstream, and it acts as an antistress agent in helping to calm tension. Pantothenic acid is found in royal honeybee jelly, raw mushrooms, broccoli, cauliflower, egg yolk, and brewer's yeast and in such common foods as organ meats, peanuts, whole grains, and beans.

Are the B vitamins involved in cancer prevention?

As early as 1944, scientists were investigating the potential of folic acid, a B vitamin, to inhibit cancer development. More recently, C. E. Butterworth and coworkers have shown that folic acid (folate) plays a key role in the maturation and differentiation of normal cells. Butterworth and his colleagues gave oral folic acid or a vitamin C placebo daily for 3 months to forty-seven women with mild or moderate cervical dysplasia while the women continued their use of combination-type oral contraceptives. Significant improvement in the tissue slides was observed in the folic acid-treated group compared with the placebo group, which showed no change, suggesting that folic acid may prevent the progression of precancerous lesions and may in some cases promote a reversal to normalcy.

Joseph Chu of the Fred Hutchinson Cancer Research Center in Seattle is studying the effect of oral folic acid as a chemopreventive agent in women at high risk of developing cervical cancer. Women will receive daily either folic acid or a similar-appearing placebo. They will be examined every 3 months for a minimum of 12 months. The regression and progression rates of cervical dysplasia will be measured. Blood samples from all patients will also be analyzed for serum folate, vitamin A, beta carotene, vitamin C, vitamin E, and antibody levels for sexually transmitted organisms. In addition, a detailed interview will focus on gynecologic history, dietary and vitamin intake, and personal habits.

What role does vitamin C play in the human body?

Vitamin C stimulates the immune system so that resistance to disease is improved. It is needed to protect the brain and spinal cord, for collagen synthesis, to manufacture neurotransmitters, and for lipid and carbohydrate metabolism.

Do all mammals need vitamin C?

Yes, all mammals need it—and all except humans, apes, guinea pigs, and fruit-eating bats manufacture it. In fact, when comparing humans with animals such as goats and dogs, it is interesting to note that these animals produce about 10 grams of vitamin C per 150 pounds of weight, and more under stressful conditions. (The FDA recommends a daily allowance of vitamin C for humans of .06 gram, or 60 milligrams.)

Why does scurvy result in people who take large amounts of vitamin C and then stop?

The reason is unknown, but scurvy, a classic sign of vitamin C deficiency, has been diagnosed in people who had been taking huge amounts of vitamin C and suddenly stopped. Dependency and withdrawal reactions have been described in people who grew accustomed to daily doses of vitamin C as low as 200 milligrams. So-called "rebound scurvy" has been reported after withdrawal from heavy doses of vitamin C. Individuals who received extra vitamin C during the siege of Leningrad had an increased incidence of scurvy when the siege was lifted and they returned to their normal diets. There are also reports of scurvy in infants of mothers who took high doses of vitamin C during pregnancy.

What major studies have been done on vitamin C and cancer prevention?

Laboratory and animal research shows that both vitamins C and E block the formation of nitrosamines. In some studies large doses of vitamin C have completely protected rats against chemically induced liver tumors and have partially protected them from lung and kidney tumors.

Epidemiologic studies suggest that fruits and vegetables containing vitamin C may offer specific protection for the upper digestive tract. Studies in northern Iran suggest that diets low in fruits and vegetables may be responsible for the high incidence there of cancers of the esophagus and, more specifically, that diets very low in fresh fruits and vegetables may in fact *contribute* to cancer of the esophagus. Japanese who eat yellow and green vegetables daily appear to have a lower risk of lung cancer, regardless of whether they are smokers or nonsmokers, than people who rarely eat these foods. There are several other similar preliminary studies that have suggested the need for further trials.

Basil C. Morson and coworkers at St. Mark's Hospital in London, in collaboration with Jerome DeCosse of Memorial Sloan-Kettering Cancer Center in New York, have reported the results of a human study to examine the potential use of vitamin C in preventing cancer of the large bowel. Patients with familial polyposis, an inherited disorder characterized by polyps, were given either large oral doses of vitamin C or a placebo. The trend toward reduction of rectal polyps in the vitamin C-treated group suggested a need for further studies of this effect, several of which are now under way.

Roy Shore of the New York University Medical Center is conducting a 3-year study to investigate the role of dietary factors—including vitamins A, C, and E, beta carotene, selenium, and protease inhibitors (which prevent the breakdown of proteins into smaller units) as well as fats and fibers—in inhibiting cancer of the colon and rectum.

Steven Tannenbaum of MIT is evaluating various dietary factors that may prevent nitrosamine formation. Healthy volunteers are receiving 2 grams of vitamin C daily; nitrosamine formation is being measured. A similar trial using 7 to 15 milligrams of vitamin E daily is in progress.

T. Colacchio of Dartmouth is conducting pilot studies to obtain sufficient information to develop a clinical trial with vitamins C and E as dietary supplements for persons at high risk for colon cancer.

W. R. Bruce and colleagues at the Ludwig Institute for Cancer Research in Toronto are conducting a double-blind study to evaluate the protective effects of vitamins C and E in lowering the recurrence rate of colon polyps; half the patients receive a placebo and the other half a combination of vitamins C and E.

If vitamin C, vitamin A, and beta carotene help reduce cancer risk, why not simply buy them in pill form from the drugstore or the health food store?
The most we presently know about the role of vitamins in cancer prevention is that populations that had low incidences of some types of cancer ate foods known to be high in those vitamins. It

is not certain, however, whether the low cancer incidence is due to vitamin intake per se or whether the foods contain other unidentified substances, such as micronutrients, that are responsible for the effect. Also, high doses of some vitamins, like vitamin A, are toxic. That is why you should eat fresh dark-green and deep-yellow vegetables and deep-yellow fruits, which are rich sources of fiber as well as carotenes (precursors of vitamin A) and vitamin C. Whole-grain products are a good source of fiber and vitamin E. Cruciferous vegetables—a group comprised of cabbage, brussels sprouts, broccoli, cauliflower, kale, and turnips—appear to contain substances that help strengthen the body's defenses against some chemical carcinogens.

Is the sun a good source of vitamin D?

Yes. The hot, steaming sun in summer is the best source of vitamin D, an important vitamin because it helps calcium to be absorbed by the intestinal wall and to be deposited in the bones. People who live in northern cities are especially vulnerable in the winter, with the weaker sunlight. The elderly, many of whom do not get outdoors often enough to benefit from the sun's rays, may need to build up their vitamin D supplies, either from food (cod, sardines, herring, liver, and egg yolks are highest in vitamin D) or from a supplement. The recommended daily allowance is 400 international units (IU). Vitamin D is stored in the body, and too much can cause problems.

What studies are being done on vitamin E and cancer prevention?

Vitamin E has been reported to reduce the incidence of chemically induced tumors of the colon in mice, but epidemiologic data concerning the protective effect of vitamin E on cancer are scarce.

In 1965, A. A. Abrams reported that vitamin E is effective in reducing the clinical symptoms of fibrocystic disease of the breast—that is, the lumpiness, size, and number of cysts, pain, and tenderness. Seven years later, Robert S. London and coworkers at Sinai Hospital in Baltimore, Maryland, showed that this clinical response was correlated with changes in the concentrations of certain steroid hormones that are excreted in the urine. In 1978, Dr. London's laboratory showed that the clinical improvement in 75 percent of a small group of patients with fibrocystic disease of the breast was correlated with steroid concentrations in both serum and urine, as well as lipid concentration changes in the serum. The NCI states that the relevance of these studies to breast cancer is unknown at this time.

Can vitamins C and E prevent cancer?

Animal studies have shown that agents such as vitamins C and E may prevent, inhibit, or reverse carcinogenesis. Vitamin C (ascorbic acid) is abundant in citrus fruits, tomatoes, and certain vegetables. Vitamin E (alpha tocopherol) is found in vegetable oils, whole grains, liver, beans, fruits, and vegetables.

Vitamins C and E appear to prevent the formation of nitrosamines, potential carcinogens that result from reactions in the digestive tract of nitrates, nitrites, and substances readily found in foods. Nitrites include nitrite salts added to meat for color, flavor development, and control of bacterial contamination; nitrate salts used in food processing that are reduced to nitrite in the body; and nitrogen oxides derived from the "smoking" process. Nitrites react with amines or amides in the digestive tract to form nitrosamines and nitrosamides. Fermentation processes, such as pickling or brewing, permit conversion of a variety of nitrogen sources, including ammonia and amino acids, to nitrite. Vitamins C and E compete with the amine or amide for the nitrosating agent. If the vitamin "wins," reacting with the nitrosating agent, the formation of nitrosamines and nitrosamides is blocked.

Can vitamins help prevent lung cancer?

Several studies are following up on the theory that vitamins can prevent lung cancer:

Gilbert S. Omenn of the Fred Hutchinson Cancer Research Center in Seattle is recruiting persons occupationally exposed to asbestos who are at high risk for lung cancer and mesothelioma for a study of the cancer-prevention effect of daily oral beta carotene and retinol (vitamin A).

Gary Goodman, also at Fred Hutchinson, is conducting studies on cigarette smokers or discontinued smokers between the ages of 50 and 65. During a 2-year pilot study, patients will receive either retinol, beta carotene, a combination of the two, or a placebo. Experience gained in the pilot will help develop a study of some 12,000 to 15,000 people who will receive either some form of vitamin A or beta carotene, depending on the results of the pilot study. The study groups will be monitored for occurrence of lung cancer.

Jussi Huttunen and Olli Heinonen of the National Public Health Institute of Helsinki, Finland, are comparing the effect of oral synthetic beta carotene and vitamin E, separately and in combination, versus placebo, in reducing the cases of lung cancer among some 19,000 male smokers between the ages of 55 and 69 at high risk for lung cancer.

Carlos L. Krumdieck of the University of Alabama is studying whether vitamin B_{12} and folate (a type of vitamin B) supplements will reduce cases of lung cancer among some 115 men between the ages of 45 and 65 who have smoked at least one pack of cigarettes a day for 20 years and have an abnormal sputum smear.

Oncologist Gabriel Gasic at Pennsylvania Hospital in Philadelphia is experimenting with an extract from the saliva of the South American leech. He has discovered that, when injected into mice with lung cancer, the extract keeps tumors from spreading. It appears that there is an active anticoagulant in the saliva that prevents blood clots—which are believed to be nesting places for circulating tumor cells. Leeches are also sometimes used by surgeons in reattaching severed fingers. When applied to the area being attached, the leech draws off excess blood and prevents obstructive blood clots.

Can calcium help prevent colon cancer?

Research conducted at Memorial Sloan-Kettering Cancer Center in New York City provides biological evidence that people may be able to lower the risk of colon cancer by adding calcium to the diet. It has been shown that calcium binds to bile acids and fatty acids, inactivating them and preventing them from acting on the cells of the colon. The study was conducted on a group of people who had family histories of colon cancers. Before the people took the calcium, the cells in the linings of their colons were producing new cells at a relatively high rate, a condition associated with a high risk of colon cancer. After a course of calcium supplements of about 1800 milligrams per day, the colon linings were producing cells at a much slower rate, comparable with those of Seventh-Day Adventists, who are largely vegetarians and have a very low rate of colon cancer.

Is there any evidence that the combination of vitamin D plus calcium is related to prevention of colorectal cancer?
Cedric Garland and his colleagues at the University of California, San Diego, studied nearly 2000 men employed by the Western Electric Company. Nutritionists compiled 28-day dietary histories during the first examination of participants and again 1 year later. Information on new cases of cancer in these men was obtained over the next 19 years. Garland and his associates found that the forty-nine men who developed colorectal cancer had a significantly lower dietary intake of vitamin D and calcium than the rest of the group. This was true even after the researchers accounted for weight, cigarette use, alcohol consumption, age, and percent of calories obtained from fat.

The study is a follow-up to research done by Garland and his brother, Frank Garland, which showed that geographic areas in the United States that gets less natural sunlight have higher death rates from colon cancer. States like California, Arizona, and New Mexico, which have high average levels of sunlight, have much lower rates of colon cancer than states like New York, New Hampshire, and Vermont. Since sunlight is a primary source of vitamin D, Garland felt that dietary as well as sunlight-produced vitamin D may have a protective effect against colon cancer. The study shows that the men who had the lowest dietary intake of vitamin D and calcium had a colorectal cancer rate of 38.9 per thousand, while in the group with the highest rate of consumption the risk was 14.3 per thousand, based on the 19-year period of observation.

Besides vitamin D plus calcium, what vitamins may have a role in preventing colorectal cancer?
There are several studies under way to research this question. Jerome DeCosse, at Memorial Sloan-Kettering Cancer Center in New York City, is assessing the effect of dietary intake of vitamin C and vitamin E together or combined with wheat fiber on precancerous rectal growths in patients who have previously undergone colorectal surgery.

Phyllis Bowen of the University of Illinois at Chicago is con-

ducting studies to see if people with low vitamin A intake and/
or marginal vitamin A levels in their blood have an increased risk
of developing colon polyps and/or colon cancer. She is also re-
searching whether beta carotene reduces the risk of colon cancer
in these patients or in patients with less severe forms of colon
polyps.

Robert Greenberg of Dartmouth College in New Hampshire is
giving some 1200 patients daily supplements of beta carotene
and/or vitamins C and E to see if either can prevent colon polyps
in people at high risk.

**Are vitamins being studied in relation to cancer of the esoph-
agus?**
Lin County in China, a rural area with a high incidence of cancer
of the esophagus, is the locale for studying the potential of multiple vitamins and minerals to prevent this cancer. There are approximately three new cases of esophageal cancer diagnosed each
day among the 700,000 people in this population, compared with
one new case each *month* among whites in a comparable U.S.
population.

Some 3000 men and women, between 40 and 69 years old,
who have abnormal cells in their esophagi (confirmed by microscopic exams), will be taking either a combination of vitamins
and minerals (comprised of vitamins A, B_2, B_6, C, and E; beta
carotene; and selenium, zinc, and molybdenum) or a placebo. In
another study, some 30,000 men and women, also between 40
and 69, will be taking either a lower dose of the vitamin-mineral
combination, one of six combinations consisting of two to three
vitamins from the complete set, or a placebo.

**What vitamin research is being done on cervical cancer pre-
vention?**
Studies to see if forms of vitamin A (retinoids) will prevent or
delay the beginning of cervical cancer in women who have
abnormal cervical cells (moderate or severe dysplasia) and are
at high risk of developing cervical cancer are now in progress.
Frank L. Meyskens and Earl Surwit of the University of Arizona Health Sciences Center in Tucson are conducting research
among 300 women with mild to moderate cervical dysplasia
by using retinoic acid in a cream form and a collagen sponge

within a cervical cap. Seymour Romney at the Albert Einstein College of Medicine in New York City is testing retinyl acetate dissolved in a gel and applied to the cervix with a vaginal applicator. Joseph Chu's research using oral folic acid at the Fred Hutchinson Cancer Research Center in Seattle is discussed on page 86.

Did our early ancestors have vitamin deficiencies?

In spite of the fact that they ate from a limited supply of available food, primitive societies appear to have been quite healthy, although their age span was short. They ate nuts, fruits, vegetables, and the lean meat of wild animals. Salt was unavailable, as was sugar. In a classic study of African bushmen, a blood cholesterol level just over half of that of Western man was found and virtually no vitamin deficiencies seemed to exist. Our nutritional patterns differ sharply from the habits evolved by humans through hundreds of thousands of generations.

Minerals

Are trace minerals important to the immune system?

It has been suggested that life evolved because of the unique electrochemical properties of metals in specific reducing or oxidizing environments. Because both epidemiologic and animal studies regarding zinc and other trace minerals such as copper, molybdenum, and iodine are limited, the connection between dietary and nutritional status and the functioning of the immune system has not been fully explored and documented. The close and sometimes diametrically opposite conclusions of the relationships between zinc and iron, zinc and copper, as well as the involvement and interactions of selenium, cadmium, and other trace elements, indicate that there is still a great deal of mystery involved with the study of trace minerals, immune function, and immune diseases. One thing is certain: to ignore the role that trace elements play in this area is to ignore the history of man and eons of biochemical evolution.

Why is chromium important to the immune system?

Chromium is a mineral contained in minute but vital quantities throughout our bodies. The immune system has a special need for chromium in white blood cells, and stress can deplete the chromium supply in those cells. There is evidence that one contributing factor in the development of blood-sugar disorders is an imbalance or malfunction of the chromium-insulin mechanism. In some experiments with chromium therapy, diabetic adults were able to function normally again after only a few months. Whole wheat flour, brewer's yeast, nuts, black pepper, whole-grain cereals (except rye and corn), fresh fruit juices, dairy products, seafood, chicken, root vegetables, legumes, leafy vegetables, and mushrooms all contain chromium. Taking 2 tablespoons of brewer's yeast daily is an excellent way to ensure an adequate supply of chromium—as well as other trace minerals—in your diet.

Why is iodine important to the immune system?

Iodine is an important mineral because it is involved in the thyroid gland's production of the vital hormone thyroxine. Adequate thyroxine is necessary in order for vitamin A to be properly synthesized from the carotene in our diets. Since vitamin A is vital to the immune system, an iodine deficiency may be at the heart of lowered resistance. Egg yolks, dairy products, brewer's yeast, wheat germ, tofu, and bean sprouts are good sources of iodine.

Does iron have a role in the immune system?

Iron deficiency can impair the immune system, making a person more susceptible to colds and infections. Iron deficiency occurs in two stages. At first, when there is a lack of iron, the body—which needs iron to produce oxygen-bearing hemoglobin—gets it from iron stored in the liver, spleen, and bone marrow. When that is gone, the body can't make enough hemoglobin, and anemia results. The symptoms of anemia are tiredness, shortness of breath, and paleness.

The recommended daily allowance of iron for women of childbearing age is 18 milligrams; for a man it is 10 milligrams. A woman needs more iron than a man because she loses some during menstruation each month. Pregnant or breastfeeding women need about double the amount. Children need more than men because they are growing. Be careful not to overdose on iron-supplement pills, because too much iron can be dangerous.

You get iron from the food you eat, but much of the iron is lost. The body absorbs iron from meat more easily than from other foods. Here are some suggestions for mixing foods to get the most iron out of them:

- Eat or drink foods high in iron such as dried prunes, dates, raisins, beans (navy, soy, red kidney), black walnuts, roasted almonds, bran flakes, oysters, cooked greens, and tomato juice.
- Eat or drink foods high in vitamin C (orange juice, broccoli) with foods that are high in iron.
- Eat 1 to 3 ounces of meat or fish when you have other iron-rich foods.
- Don't drink tea or coffee with your meal; it can reduce the absorption of iron-rich foods.

How does magnesium work?

Magnesium is necessary to the life of every cell in the body. It is needed by cells to produce proteins to replenish and replace themselves. It is one of the body's most important coenzymes, a helper in the numerous biochemical processes catalyzed by enzymes in the cell. When the immune system is attacked by bacteria or viruses, magnesium swings into action with a blood protein (properdin) to put an end to the invaders. Magnesium is found in most unadulterated foods, so it is not difficult to get an adequate supply in the diet. Nuts and seeds, kale, endive, beet greens, alfalfa sprouts, and celery are all high in magnesium.

What is the value of potassium?

Potassium is an important trace element that can be depleted in the bodily system by vomiting, diarrhea, or the overuse of diuretics. Low potassium levels have an injurious effect on the heart and other muscles. Potassium is most abundant in lima beans, watermelon, spinach, artichokes, potatoes, brussels sprouts, broccoli, bananas, carrots, and celery.

Are there known potassium depleters?

Licorice is known to deplete potassium levels. Therefore, since licorice is an additive widely used in tobacco products, it is thought that licorice may be a contributing factor in the high cancer rate among smokers.

What vitamins can help to increase potassium levels?

Both vitamins A and C have been found to increase the intracellular potassium-sodium ratio. Low cancer rates have been associated with high-fiber vegetables and fruits that are high in potassium and low in sodium.

What research has been done on potassium intake and cancer?

According to a 10-year study at the University of Texas, M.D. Anderson Hospital and Tumor Institute, led by Birger Jansson, Ph.D., high potassium intake can significantly decrease a person's cancer risk. The study was undertaken to determine why there is a low colorectal cancer rate in Seneca County, New York, in spite of the fact that the area is located in a region that has the highest colorectal cancer rate in the nation. The unique geochemical makeup of Seneca County was found to be the most probable explanation for its low rate of colorectal cancer. Seneca's drinking water comes from two deep glacial lakes that penetrate the underlying salt strata, causing the sum of the concentrations of high potassium and low sodium salts to be between ten and twenty times that of other lakes in the state. In correlating information, it was noted that Utah (the Great Salt Lake area) has the lowest cancer rates in the United States. The potassium salts concentration in this lake was found to be even higher than in Seneca's lakes, and the potassium-sodium ratio three times higher than that of the lakes at Seneca.

What does selenium do?

Selenium forms a part of large enzyme molecules. Its primary role is as an antioxidant, preventing breakdown of fats and other body chemicals. It is known to interact with vitamin E. Studies have shown that in areas where selenium is available in low amounts in water and soil, there are higher cancer rates and more deaths from high blood pressure. A study in mice shows that when selenium is added to drinking water, the incidence of breast cancer and precancerous colon tumors is reduced. When given to animals before the development of cancer cells by viral or chemical means, selenium appears to prevent the onset of cancer. It must be noted, however, that selenium has not succeeded in inhibiting the growth rate of tumors that were already established.

Are there any studies that show whether or not selenium might prevent cancer?

There are both laboratory and animal studies indicating that certain forms of selenium (found in seafood, organ meats, and grains, especially those grown in some geographic areas) may possibly prevent cancer. Carmia Borek of Columbia University has reported that selenium may "protect" against radiation- and chemical-induced cancer in cells grown in the laboratory. The incidence of chemically induced colon cancer and liver tumors in rats can be reduced by adding certain forms of selenium to the drinking water.

There is also epidemiologic evidence on the relationship between selenium and cancer from a number of geographical correlation studies that associate cancer risk with estimates of individual selenium intake, with levels of selenium in the blood, or with selenium concentrations in the water supply or soil. In the northeastern United States, high rates of colon, rectal, and breast cancer have been correlated with industrialization, high intake of dietary fat, and low levels of selenium in the soil. According to the National Cancer Institute, in most areas studied there is an inverse relationship between selenium level and cancer. However, whether this is a cause-effect relationship cannot be determined because of confounding effects such as industrialization. Moreover, it is not clear whether this relationship applies to all cancer sites or only to specific ones, such as the digestive tract. Data related to selenium intake are being gathered now in studies in China, Finland, and other countries on people who are receiving selenium supplements or have low selenium intakes. In addition, the National Cancer Institute is funding several studies with selenium.

What are some of the trials on selenium that the National Cancer Institute is sponsoring?

Charles Hennekens and his coworkers at Brigham and Women's Hospitals in Boston are conducting a pilot study to determine the feasibility of a trial of selenium, a form of vitamin A, and vitamin E as chemopreventive agents against cancer in a population of healthy volunteer dentists.

Walter Willett of the Harvard School of Public Health is studying whether persons with low levels of dietary selenium are at increased risk of developing cancer of the breast, lung, and large bowel.

Frank Polk at Johns Hopkins University in Baltimore is relating the levels of various serum constituents (antioxidant vitamins including retinol-binding protein, vitamin E, and beta carotene;

selenium; hormones; and antibodies to cytomegalovirus and Epstein-Barr virus) to the subsequent occurrence of cancer.

The National Cancer Institute and the U.S. Department of Agriculture have studies to gain information about the body's response to, dietary assessment of, interactions of, and measurements of certain nutrients. In an early study, healthy volunteers are receiving a single dose and a prolonged dose of selenium, with researchers examining the blood levels and body responses with respect to both the organic and inorganic forms of selenium. A similar pilot study will be done with beta carotene.

What is known about our need for zinc?
Zinc is required for both DNA and RNA synthesis. Many studies show that a deficiency in zinc weakens the ability of thymidine to be incorporated into DNA and adversely affects all the steps occurring in a reproducing cell population. Several enzymes involved in RNA and DNA synthesis seem to require zinc.

Have the effects of zinc been studied in healthy individuals?
Duchateau and colleagues in Brussels have conducted research showing that zinc supplementation may have a regulatory effect on the immune systems of normal, healthy individuals. Eighty-three persons, all healthy adults (young men; young and older women, some taking oral contraceptives), were given daily supplements of zinc. Another group of individuals was studied but not given the supplements. After a month of taking the zinc, all eighty-three persons in the zinc-taking group showed an increase in lymphocyte responses.

What foods are high in zinc?
Lobster and deep-sea fish contain the highest amounts of zinc per milligram. Soy meal, wheat bran, black-eyed peas, crab, oysters, beef, lamb, dark turkey meat, and organ meats all contain high levels of zinc. Zinc can also be obtained in pill or liquid form.

How does zinc relate to selenium?
Animal studies have shown that if 200 parts per million of zinc are available in water, small amounts of selenium uptake are prevented in the face of these high zinc levels. This indicates that high levels of zinc block the effects of selenium.

Can taking too much zinc be harmful?

The Journal of the American Medical Association carried a report suggesting that taking large amounts of zinc above the recommended daily allowance can lead to significant and dangerous body changes. It can impair the body's immune response and result in changes in blood fat levels that could be potentially dangerous.

What are free radicals?

Free radicals are by-products of normal chemical reactions in your body that can make a cell develop into a cancer if not destroyed. Free radicals are also increased by harmful chemicals known to cause cancer. However, the body has natural protection against free radicals thanks to certain vitamins and minerals called antioxidants, which serve as free-radical scavengers. Carotene, vitamin E, vitamin C, zinc, selenium, and copper are potent antioxidants.

How do free radicals alter cells?

Carcinogens such as X rays and sunlight are associated with free-radical reactions capable of altering the cell's DNA. These chemical changes in the DNA alter the cell's normal regulation and may be related to cancer development. Some chemical carcinogens enter the body in an active form. Others, which are inactive when they enter, may be converted into active forms by the normal processes of various organs or by combining with other chemicals in the digestive tract. For example, nitrates can combine in the stomach with amines to form nitrosamines or with amides to form nitrosamides. This combining does not take place when some antioxidants, especially vitamin C, are present. Animal studies have shown that agents such as beta carotene, vitamin A, vitamin C, vitamin E, and the trace element selenium may prevent, inhibit, or reverse carcinogenesis—possibly by blocking free-radical reactions at the molecular level. Whether nitrosamides and nitrosamines are significant carcinogens in humans is still being debated.

What are some dietary guidelines to ensure adequate intake of vitamins and minerals?

- Stick with natural, unadulterated foods whenever possible. Whole fresh fruit and raw vegetables are better than canned or bottled.

- Bran—even just a few tablespoons a day—is essential for promoting a healthy digestive tract.
- Include yogurt in your diet. It facilitates digestion and increases resistance to infections.
- Soybean sprouts help build energy. The enzyme invertase in soybean sprouts helps convert an impoverished diet into carbohydrates.
- Wheat germ contains vitamin E, B vitamins, and important trace minerals.
- Honey contains the ten essential amino acids as well as valuable minerals: copper, iron, calcium, sodium, titanium, and potassium.
- Nutritional (brewer's) yeast contains all B vitamins in natural form.
- Even critics of vitamin megadoses agree that illnesses and infections increase the body's needs for vitamins and minerals—so a basic vitamin supplement is a good idea.

The gastrointestinal system handles between 100 and 200 tons of food during the average lifetime of a human being.

VITAMINS

	ROLE IN BODY	FOOD SOURCES
Vitamin A (fat-soluble)	Necessary for cellular differentiation. Correlates with low cancer rates; may reverse precancer states.	Liver, carrots, leafy green and yellow vegetables, raw hot chili peppers, cantaloupe, butter.
Vitamin B_1 (thiamine) (water-soluble)	Enhances immune system; releases energy from carbohydrates.	Pork, liver, oysters, whole-grain cereals, pasta and bread, brewer's yeast.
Vitamin B_2 (riboflavin) (water-soluble)	Enhances immune system; important in carbohydrate metabolism.	Liver, milk, whole grains, dark-green vegetables, mushrooms, soy.
Vitamin B_3 (niacin) (water-soluble)	Works with B_1 and B_2 in carbohydrate functions.	Liver, poultry, meat, tuna, grains, nuts, dried beans and peas.
Vitamin B_6 (pyridoxine) (water-soluble)	Enhances immune system; needed for formation of red blood cells, absorption, metabolism of proteins.	Liver, avocados, spinach, green beans, bananas, whole-grain cereals and breads.
Vitamin B_{12} (cobalamin) (water-soluble)	Necessary for genetic functions, nervous system functions, formation of red blood cells.	Liver, kidneys, eggs, milk, oysters, meat, fish, soy sauce. (Not readily available from vegetable sources.)

ADULT RECOMMENDATIONS	DEFICIENCY DANGERS AND MEGADOSE RISKS
2–3 daily servings of foods rich in vitamin A; 800–1000 mcg per day.	Deficiency dangers: night blindness, rough skin, no bone growth, dry eyes. Megadoses of 50,000 IU per day can cause dizziness, headache, and vomiting; liver, bone, and brain damage; lung cancer in men; hair loss; toxic effect involving skin and mucous membranes.
1–1.5 mg per day. Women and girls likely to be more deficient in this vitamin.	Deficiency dangers: muscular weakness, leg cramps, beriberi. Needs increase with birth-control pill use, heavy drinking.
1.2–1.7 mg per day; more needed by regular exercisers.	Deficiency can cause skin disorders, eyes oversensitive to light, lips cracked at corners.
13–20 mg per day	Deficiency can cause skin disorders (especially in parts exposed to sun), smooth tongue, diarrhea, mental confusion, pellagra. Megadose can aggravate asthma, diabetes mellitus, peptic ulcer, liver disease, gout.
2–2.2 mg per day. Need increases with increased proteins and with use of oral contraceptives, cortisone, and INH.	Deficiency can cause skin disorders (same as B_3 deficiency), nausea, anemia, kidney stones. Overdoses may cause convulsions. Symptoms of dependency seen in patients given 200 mg daily followed by withdrawal (multivitamin formula without B_6 recommended for patients with Parkinson's on L-dopa).
3–4 mcg per day. Strict vegetarians should take a B_{12} supplement.	Deficiency results in pernicious anemia, anemia, degeneration of peripheral nerves. B_{12} absorption decreases with megadoses of vitamin C.

	Role in Body	Food Sources
Folic acid (water-soluble)	Needed in formation of hemoglobin, body proteins, genetic material.	Spinach, liver, kidneys, wheat germ, brewer's yeast. Can be destroyed by cooking in copper pots.
Pantothenic acid (B₅) (water-soluble)	Enhances immune system; found in all living cells. Metabolizes carbohydrates, proteins, fats. Needed in formation of hormones and nerve-regulating substances.	Royal honeybee jelly, raw mushrooms, broccoli, cauliflower, egg yolk, brewer's yeast.
Biotin (water-soluble)	Releases energy from carbohydrates. Needed in formation of fatty acids.	Egg yolk, liver, kidneys, dark-green vegetables, green beans.
Vitamin C (ascorbic acid) (water-soluble)	Important to immune system function. Blocks formation of cancer-causing substances. Protects against infection. Maintains healthy bones, teeth, blood vessels, collagen. Antioxidant. Following surgery, illness, injury, or extensive burns, body needs for vitamin C increase.	Fruits and vegetables (especially citrus fruits and dark-green vegetables), sweet red and green peppers, potatoes.

ADULT RECOMMENDATIONS	DEFICIENCY DANGERS AND MEGADOSE RISKS
400 mcg per day; 800 mcg per day for pregnant women. Birth-control pill use or alcoholism may lead to deficiency.	Deficiencies may lead to megalo-blastic anemia, smooth tongue, diarrhea. Folic acid is stored in liver and kidney, so deficiency may result from inability to absorb. Large amounts of folic acid can mask B_{12} deficiency.
No RDA determined; 4–7 mg per day estimated as safe.	Deficiency can cause vomiting, ab-dominal pain, sleep problems. Ex-cessive consumption increases need for thiamine and may precipitate thiamine-deficiency symptoms.
No RDA determined; 100–120 mcg per day estimated as safe.	Loss of appetite, depression, fa-tigue, nausea, and pains may be re-sults of deficiency. Those who eat many raw eggs should watch for biotin deficiency. Avidin, a protein in uncooked egg white, binds the vi-tamin and prevents absorption. Cooking destroys avidin.
60–100 mg per day	Deficiency causes scurvy, bleeding gums, degeneration of muscles, slow wound healing, loosening teeth, rough skin. Megadoses may cause deficiency symptoms on re-turn to normal levels. Also, too much vitamin C causes formation of bladder and kidney stones, de-stroys B_{12} and calcium, and may al-low absorption of too much iron. Heavy smokers and women taking oral contraceptives may need more than minimum daily requirement. Excess vitamin C during pregnancy has been known to cause "re-bound" scurvy in infants and an abnormally large need for vitamin C. Elderly absorb less vitamin C than younger adults.

	ROLE IN BODY	FOOD SOURCES
Vitamin D (fat-soluble)	Essential for normal bone growth.	Sunshine vitamin. Also available in milk, egg yolk, fish.
Vitamin E (alpha tocopherol) (fat-soluble)	Essential to red blood cells, muscle, and other tissue. Has role in blocking production of nitrosamines in intestinal tract. Antioxidant.	Cottonseed oil, olive oil, walnuts, almonds, alfalfa, wheat germ, cabbage, peanuts, lettuce, popcorn.
Vitamin K (fat-soluble)	Needed for blood clotting.	Green leafy vegetables, vegetables in cabbage family, milk.

Adult Recommendations	Deficiency Dangers and Megadose Risks
10 mcg for infants, teens, women; 5 mcg for adult males; 10 mcg during pregnancy and while nursing. 10 mcg = 400 IU of vitamin D.	Deficiency causes rickets, retarded growth in children, soft bones, and muscle twitching and spasms in adults. Excessive consumption is poisonous; can cause kidney damage, lethargy, loss of appetite.
30 IU per day	Deficiency causes breakdown of red blood cells. High dosages can cause a variety of problems, including thrombophlebitis, pulmonary embolism, hypertension, vaginal bleeding, visual complaints, possible aggravation of diabetes mellitus and angina pectoris.
No RDA determined; 70–140 mcg estimated as safe. Extra K needed in adults with impaired fat absorption, cancer, or kidney disease.	Deficiency can cause hemorrhaging in newborns, those on sulfa drugs, or those with impaired fat absorption. Excessive use of vitamin K can be toxic. Prolonged use of antibiotics can destroy bacteria that normally produce vitamin K.

MINERALS

	ROLE IN BODY	FOOD SOURCES
Calcium	Most abundant mineral in body. Plays role in blood coagulation as well as normal functioning of nerves, muscles, heartbeat.	Milk, milk products, dark-green and leafy vegetables.
Iron	Necessary for transport of oxygen to tissues and for cellular oxidation functions.	Liver, red meats, dried beans and peas, whole-grain breads, cereals.
Selenium	Believed to be associated with vitamin E in its functions; prevents breakdown of fats and other body chemicals.	Garlic, wheat germ, seafood, egg yolk, chicken, whole grains, milk, meat.
Zinc	Necessary for protein synthesis and cell division.	Red meat, milk, liver, seafood, eggs, whole grains.
Potassium	Intracellular fluid controls activity of heart muscles, nervous system, kidneys.	Bananas, cantaloupes, apricots, wheat germ, green vegetables, raisins, sunflower seeds.

ADULT RECOMMENDATIONS	DEFICIENCY DANGERS AND MEGADOSE RISKS
800–1500 mg per day	Overdoses can cause drowsiness and impaired absorption of other minerals.
18 mg per day	Depletion of iron may result in anemia. Overdose may cause toxic buildup in liver, pancreas, and heart.
.05 to .2 mg per day	Megadoses may cause nausea; loss of hair, fingernails, and toenails. Selenium supplements can be toxic, and overdoses cause death in animals.
15 mg per day	Deficiency associated with anemia, short stature, impaired wound healing. Overdoses can cause nausea, vomiting, premature birth, stillbirth.
No RDA determined; 2000–2500 mg estimated as safe	Deficiency associated with giddiness and confusion, weakening of heart and other muscles. Deficiency may follow vomiting and diarrhea or use of diuretics.

chapter 4

New Ways of
Strengthening Immunity

The medical literature of the past 5 years is full of an emerging science with unlimited potential for strengthening immunity. New methods being tested in scientific laboratories throughout the world have yielded a host of new techniques that have made gene therapy, monoclonal antibodies, interferon, and antirejection compounds a new frontier in the treatment of diseases such as cancer, AIDS, and herpes. They hold promise for alleviating many other immune system disorders as well. Better understanding of the role of DNA has flung open the doors to new possibilities in manipulating genes in disease therapy. This exciting and rapidly changing field is causing a revolution in the way medical science is treating many of the most resistant diseases of humankind.

Gene Therapy

What are genes?
Genes govern the traits we inherit from our fathers and mothers and from the generations before them. They tell the body's cells how to manufacture particular proteins. Genes are contained in the DNA—a long strand of materials that comprises the body's inner map of development.

How many genes are there in the body?
The number is staggering. Every human cell contains about 100,000 genes. These genes, taken together, contain some 6 billion nucleotides; a nucleotide is a single pair of nucleic acids,

either adenine-thymine (A-T) or cytosine-guanine (C-G). When strung together up to hundreds of thousands of times, these nucleotides "write" the genes' message. Each cell in the body contains the same genetic information, this code made up of tens of thousands of genes. All 6 billion nucleotides are present in each of the 100 trillion cells in the body.

A defect in a single gene can cause painful, devastating illness or certain, early death. Scientists have isolated 21,500 of the 100,000 genes and identified the specific jobs they do in the body. They know, for instance, the chemical structure of the gene that makes insulin, a hormone which, when lacking, causes diabetes.

What is DNA?

DNA (for deoxyribonucleic acid, the chemical name for the genetic code) is found in every cell of the body. DNA, a strand 2 yards long, contains the code made up of a four-letter alphabet that gives the body instructions. When cells divide, the DNA duplicates itself and passes along its genetic code to the next generation of cells. DNA directs the assembly of amino acids into the proteins essential for normal functioning of the body.

The DNA resembles a spiral ladder or double helix, with the rungs made up of pairs of four nucleotide bases: adenine (A), guanine (G), cytosine (C), and thymine (T). In forming a rung, A always pairs with T, and G always pairs with C. This sequence of nucleotides along one strand of DNA comprises the code that dictates the assembly of a protein. Because proteins are long and complex, the blueprint for one may consist of thousands of A's, T's, G's, and C's, all arranged in a precise order. In genetic diseases, the order somehow gets mixed up. In sickle-cell anemia, for instance, a T is located in the DNA ladder where an A is supposed to be. Researchers are now able to decipher the DNA code and find errors in the coding.

What are enhancers?

Enhancers are part of the DNA. Researchers believe that enhancers may tell the cell to make more of a product necessary to meet the body's demand. If, for example, the body has to metabolize more sugars, it may be the enhancer that tells the insulin-producing cells to make more insulin. Enhancers—which have also been called activators, augmenters, and potentiators by different researchers—may be one of the mechanisms that switches the genes that code for the products the body needs into greater expression.

Only 30 Years of DNA Knowledge

It was in 1953 in Cambridge, England, that two young men, James D. Watson and Francis H.C. Crick, discovered the structure of the master chemical of heredity of all living things. In a brief letter published in the April 25, 1953, issue of the scientific journal *Nature*, they revealed to the world the soon-to-be-famous double-helix structure of DNA. The structure showed scientists how the chemical code of life was organized and might be deciphered. Although DNA itself was discovered in 1969, it was the 1953 discovery of the double-helix structure that opened new doors in research around the world. Many scientists call it the century's most important medical scientific discovery. Watson, Crick, and their colleague, Maurice H.F. Wilkins, were awarded the Nobel Prize in physiology and medicine in 1962.

How do enhancers work?
Scientists do not yet know how enhancers work. Several possibilities have been proposed, but they are all still theories. All of them may be correct.

- The enhancers may alter the shape of chromatin (DNA and proteins), perhaps opening it up slightly, allowing transcription—the process of moving information from the DNA to other parts of the cell—to occur.
- The enhancers may keep protective proteins surrounding the DNA away from specific genes.
- The enhancer may contain some nucleotides that bind the chromosome—very long strands of DNA—to an area of the cellular nucleus where transcription can occur more easily.

The mechanism by which enhancers work has become one of the most actively pursued scientific questions. Researchers feel that its answer may provide an insight into the areas of cell development and control as well as into the diseases that result from defects in normal regulation.

On what genetic diseases is scientific research focusing?

Presently, with the limited understanding scientists have of gene therapy, three rare diseases—all caused by the failure of a single defective gene to produce a single crucial enzyme—are being targeted. The diseases are Lesch-Nyhan disease, which damages the kidneys and also produces mental retardation, and ADA deficiency and PNP deficiency, both of which cause the immune system to collapse, with patients dying in childhood of overwhelming infection.

There are between 2000 and 3000 known inherited diseases, but most of them are too complex to be unraveled with today's limited knowledge of gene structure. Researchers believe that within 5 years most of the genes causing genetic diseases will have been either isolated or identified by markers and that DNA probes for precise diagnosis of many will be available. Eventually, it may be possible to provide genetic profiles, so that preventive steps can be taken. A person with genes for skin cancer would be alerted to use sun blocks, for instance.

What are gene probes?

Presently in the experimental stages, gene probes are synthetically created single strands of DNA that are designed from genes linked to diseases. When put into a patient's tissue or fluid sample, the probe will comb the cells for their complementary halves—other single strands of DNA. Tagged with a radioactive or fluorescent material, the probes will send up a flare when they bond with their counterparts—showing scientists where the problem gene is on the cell. Probes will eventually be able, for example, to accurately single out genes for heart disease so that the person can make preventive modifications in his or her lifestyle. More than 750 gene probes have been designed for laboratory research into genetically linked diseases including sickle-cell anemia, muscular dystrophy, hemophilia, and Lesch-Nyhan syndrome.

What is a retrovirus?

A retrovirus is a special kind of virus, so named because instead of reproducing in the ordinary way, it copies its genes backwards. This backwardness gives retroviruses an ability to infect their targets in a devastating way; an example is the AIDS virus. However, scientists believe that the ability of the virus to inject its genes into the host cell's genes can be used in a positive way.

Scientists plan to use retroviruses to put a good gene into the human body to do the work of a defective gene. They will take a virus incapable of causing infection or tumors, put a human gene into it, and then inject the altered virus into the body. Although altered, the virus is still capable of slipping inside a cell and delivering its genetic material to the cell's nucleus. But instead of its own genetic material, the virus inserts a human gene into the host cell's DNA. The new gene can override the inborn error that causes a genetic disease.

So far gene therapy has been limited to experiments in mice and monkeys, with a few trials on white blood cells in laboratory test tubes. In the not too distant future, researchers will be injecting the altered viruses into humans, with the first candidate being an infant with ADA deficiency.

Is there work with gene therapy in the cancer field?
Yes, there is. Most cancer researchers believe that somehow, usually over a long period of years, carcinogens repeatedly brought into the body finally damage a critical piece of a cell's code. The damage causes it to send out abnormal messages related to some aspect of cell growth. As new cells spring from old, the misled cell leads to an onslaught of others that result in runaway growth. Eventually the altered growth genes, known as oncogenes (from the Greek *onco*, meaning *tumor*), take charge. To date, nearly thirty cancer genes have been identified in experiments in animals or in normal human cells grown in the laboratory.

How do cells change from normal to cancerous?
Scientists believe that most cancer develops in at least two steps, by two kinds of agents: initiators and promoters. *Initiators* start the damage to the cell, damage that can lead to cancer. For example, cigarette smoking, X rays, and certain chemicals have been shown to be initiators. *Promoters* stimulate the development of cancer but usually do not by themselves cause cancer. They change the cells already damaged by the initiator from normal cells to cancerous cells. Research has shown that alcohol promotes the development of cancer in the mouth, throat, and possibly liver when combined with an initiator such as tobacco. Alcohol is a classic example of a promoter: It alone does not cause cancer, but it is clearly associated with cancer's causation.

Where have oncogenes been found?
Scientists have found versions of oncogenes in several kinds of

human cancer, including those of the breast, lung, bladder, and bowel. In addition, DNA sequences nearly identical to oncogenes have been discovered in normal tissue cells throughout the animal kingdom, including those of humans. Researchers think that such "proto-oncogenes" have existed throughout evolution and play a useful role in normal cell division. What the researchers are investigating is how these seemingly harmless genes become altered and turned into cancer genes. They have yet to unravel the mystery of what activates an oncogene, how to prevent it from turning cancerous, or, once it has turned cancerous, how to halt its perpetuation through future generations in the course of cell division.

How do oncogenes work?
Scientists believe that each of us probably carries one or more oncogenes in every cell in our body. Undisturbed, oncogenes are harmless. Then, one day, something comes along that triggers the oncogenes. They make a chemical that causes cells to divide and multiply uncontrollably, forming millions of new cells—a cancer—that invade and choke our organs.

The oncogenes start dominating the behavior of the cell. They disrupt the usual schedule and direct perpetual growth. Most researchers believe that at least two cancer genes must be created, by random error, before the process starts.

Although the role of each cancer gene is not yet understood, scientists believe that the cancerous cell growth is set off through a series of steps within the cell. Some cancer genes apparently tell the cell to overproduce a growth-factor protein or mistakenly produce an abnormal growth factor. Others may tell the cell to ignore signals to stop growing—perhaps by leaving growth-factor receptor switches on at various points along the cell's surface.

What results has oncogene research already produced?
Scientists believe that oncogene research will, in the future, lead to practical applications in diagnosis, prevention, and treatment. Already it has produced:

• ways of identifying, at the molecular level, patients who are susceptible to some cancers and those who are carriers of genetically transmitted forms of the disease, such as Wilms' tumor, a cancer that affects children;

- procedures for monitoring patients by examining sites of oncogenes on their chromosomes;
- strategies for cancer therapy, based on attacking the products of oncogenes;
- evidence that certain drugs may reverse oncogene expression.

The National Cancer Institute expects oncogene research in the next 2 years to advance quickly, due to the arrival of a supercomputer able to perform in 15 minutes experiments that now take a day to do. The computer's main function is to accelerate the basic understanding of genes, analyzing newly isolated gene sequences to determine the proteins encoded by these genes at a much faster rate than can the present computers.

What new areas of research with oncogenes are envisioned?
There are several areas. For example, research has indicated that tumor cells of lung cancer patients contain an activated oncogene not present in normal lung cells from the same patients. It is felt that this implies that change occurred as part of the beginning of the tumor and that DNA damage might have been as a result of the carcinogen in tobacco smoke. Knowing that multiple oncogenes must be activated for tumors to form may be useful in identifying smokers who may be predisposed to cancer. It may be possible in the future to look at lung cell samples for seemingly healthy smokers and determine whether a single oncogene has been activated. If so, smokers can quit before a second oncogene is activated.

Scientists also envision developing monoclonal antibodies to oncogene products for use in diagnosing and treating cancers. Monoclonal antibodies may be fitted with radioactive tracers to identify cells that are becoming cancerous at early stages and to help pinpoint small tumors. The antibodies may be used with oncogene proteins to deliver drugs directly to cancerous or potentially cancerous cells.

What happens when cells of the immune system proliferate uncontrollably?
The result of the uncontrollable proliferation of cells is cancer. Leukemias are caused by the proliferation of white blood cells, or leukocytes. The uncontrolled growth of antibody-producing (plasma) cells can lead to multiple myeloma, which affects the

bone marrow and the bones. Cancers of the lymphoid organs are called lymphomas and include Hodgkin's disease.

To what diseases besides cancer does gene therapy have applications?

Genetic engineering is bringing new hope to people afflicted with diabetes, dwarfism, and hemophilia. A person with diabetes can have an injection of a genetically engineered form of insulin that is the exact molecular duplicate of human insulin. Human growth hormone, cloned in the laboratory from human genes, is used for youngsters who are growing too slowly. Antihemophiliac factor, the substance that helps blood to clot, which hemophiliacs are missing, is now available thanks to genetic engineering.

Researchers are studying potential applications of other drugs such as endorphin, a natural morphinelike compound that controls pain and mood; human serum albumin, a protein available from blood that is used by doctors to replace blood loss from surgery or injury; streptokinase and urokinase, two enzymes that work within the blood system, dissolving blood clots in the body, particularly in the heart, brain, and lungs; and tissue plasminogen activator, a protein that dissolves blood clots, working at the site of the clot without affecting the blood supply.

Can gene-transfer techniques also be used to make the vaccines?

Yes. Splicing genes into viruses—known as gene transfer—is being used to make vaccines. Experimental vaccines have been made against herpes and hepatitis viruses. Scientists have isolated a gene from a herpes virus and transferred it into a harmless virus called vaccinia. The vaccinia was sufficiently similar to the herpes virus to stimulate the production of antibodies against herpes. When the vaccinated person was later exposed to a real herpes virus, the antibodies protected him. This same technique is used to make hepatitis vaccine.

Can doctors tell who will inherit disorders?

Scientists are learning how to pinpoint genes that cause, or predispose a person to, future illness. The process utilizes genetic probes, which contain synthetic versions of genes that cause disease. The probes are put into a test tube with a small sample of a person's own genetic material—the DNA. The probes cling to and identify their natural counterparts. In the future, probes will be able to predict diseases where there is any kind of genetic influence. Scientists are presently working on tests to detect Huntington's chorea, atherosclerosis, cancers that are known to be inherited or to have familial tendencies, and Alzheimer's disease.

Biological Response Modifiers

What are biological response modifiers?

For years scientists have searched for ways to trigger the body's own defenses against cancer. This search has led to the discovery of hundreds of biological and chemical substances that boost, direct, or restore many of the normal defenses of the body. These substances may also be useful as anticancer agents. Called "biological response modifiers," many of these substances occur naturally in the body, while others are made in the laboratory. Monoclonal antibodies are one example of a biological.

Are biological response modifiers being used to treat disease?

Biological response modifiers are in an early stage of development. Although scientists have known about them for years, isolating and purifying them so they could be used to treat diseases has been very difficult. Many of these substances occur in the body in very small amounts and may be present only for a matter of hours. New tools, such as gene-splicing, now allow scientists to produce the substances in large enough amounts so that they can be isolated, purified and studied.

Will biologicals be used in cancer treatment?

Biological response modifiers may have some roles to play in cancer treatment. They may have direct anticancer effects on some products of the body's immune system. They may also help normal body cells to control cancer cells in several ways, such as by fortifying a cancer patient's immune system so that it fights the growth of cancer cells, by eliminating or suppressing the body's responses that permit cancer growth, by making cancer cells more sensitive to being destroyed by the patient's immune system, by stimulating a cancer cell to grow and to mature into a less harmful cell or into a normal cell, by blocking the processes that change a normal cell or a precancerous cell into a cancerous cell, or by enhancing a cancer patient's ability to repair normal cells damaged by other forms of cancer treatment such as chemotherapy or radiation.

What kinds of materials are being tested to trigger the body's defenses?

The major emphasis is on agents that boost and increase the body's own immune defenses. These defenses are mostly antibodies and immune cells that help the body attack invaders such as viruses, bacteria, and possibly cancer. Certain kinds of bacteria, sugars, and synthetic agents can modify an immune response, stimulate one where none existed, or bring back a response that has been lost or used up. Some agents may also stimulate a defense against cancer cells, particularly by triggering the ''scavenger'' cells (macrophages) that devour foreign cells.

What are the names of some of the agents for triggering the body's defenses that are now being tested?

Some of the agents being tested include the following:

monoclonal antibodies
thymosin (a hormone formed by the thymus gland)
interleukin-2
interferons (synthetically produced as well as naturally occurring)

Monoclonal Antibodies

What are monocolonal antibodies?

Monoclonal antibodies are invisible bits of protein manufactured by animal and human cells grown in the test tube. Each type of antibody—and there are hundreds of them—has the incredible ability to recognize and latch onto a specific target. The target can be any living matter down to and including a single biological molecule.

Monoclonal antibodies are very small. To envision the size of a typical human cell, you need to know that 1 million would fit on the head of a pin. Compared with the size of a monoclonal antibody, a cell is huge. Grant Fjermedal in *Magic Bullets* points out that ''a monoclonal antibody sitting on a cell would be like one of the textured bumps on the surface of a basketball. So a monoclonal antibody is unimaginably small, yet that monoclonal is a whirling mass of thousands of bullets.'' The particles become increasingly smaller. The antigen is smaller than a single cell. The antibody looks tiny in relation to the antigen, and the isotope is minuscule in relation to the antibody.

What's the difference between normal antibodies and mono-clonal antibodies?

Antibodies are *natural* substances released by the immune system to fight disease. Monoclonal antibodies are broadly similar but are cultured in a test tube using some of medicine's newest technology.

Normal antibodies are Y-shaped protein molecules, produced by white blood cells, that attack any foreign matter that gets into the body. Each one precisely matches a special site on the invader's surface—be it virus, bacterium, chemical, or cell—and attacks by attaching to it in a lock-and-key fashion. This marks the foreign substance, called an antigen, and makes it a target for other cells from the immune system to recognize and destroy.

Monoclonal antibodies are produced by identical descendants, or clones, of a single cell. Their great advantage is that they can be designed to attack specific body cells, delivering lethal doses of radioactivity or toxins directly to the target, where they can attack without damaging healthy surrounding tissue. There are thousands of different monoclonals, some usable and others not. Every antibody is different, even though it might bind to the same antigen as another. The human body has the ability to code for more than a million antibodies.

In 1971, Stanley Order of Johns Hopkins University in Baltimore created polyclonal antibodies—clones from several different types of parent cells—and began doing experimental work with mice. Monoclonal antibodies, exact clones from a single parent cell, resulted from research in 1975 when Georges Kohler and Cesar Milstein of the Medical Research Council in Cambridge, England, forced antibody-making cells to fuse with cancer cells. This resulted in cells that grow like a tumor in the test tube and are known as hybridomas. The resulting cells become a microscopic antibody factory—reproducing a single type of antibody in quantities far greater than a normal cell. Hybridomas can produce antibodies by the quart. Because these antibodies come from a single clone of hybrid cells, they are called monoclonal antibodies. Practical applications of the concept of monoclonal antibodies are just beginning to be discovered.

What are some potential uses of monoclonal antibodies?
Monoclonal antibodies interact only with specific molecules in
the body and therefore can be used to pinpoint the presence of a
virus or bacterium that would otherwise escape notice. Presently
or in the future they will be used for:

- laboratory tests of unprecedented accuracy for diagnosing diseases
- treatments for cancer as well as for such intractable diseases
  as malaria and rabies
- preventing the rejection of transplanted kidneys and other organs
- identifying unknown drugs and chemicals in the body and
  treating drug overdoses
- spotting contaminants in foods and the environment
- leaching valuable chemicals out of complex solutions
- testing for pregnancy
- treating diseases such as multiple sclerosis

**What experimental work is being done with monoclonal anti-
bodies?**
At the kidney transplantation unit at Massachusetts General Hospital in Boston, monoclonal antibodies are being used to provide
early warning of transplant rejection and sometimes to halt it.
The growth of white cells (T lymphocytes), which play a role in
rejecting a transplanted organ, is tracked with monoclonals. Doctors can spot any sudden increase that would indicate a greater
risk of rejection. The transplant patients are also given a daily
shot of monoclonals for 2 weeks. The antibodies bind to the T
cells, marking them for distribution by the immune system.

At the Children's Hospital Medical Center in Boston, doctors
have used monoclonals to save the life of a week-old baby who
developed a severe reaction to a blood transfusion. Because the
child was born without a thymus gland, the baby's immune system could not neutralize the T cells in the transfused blood. Doctors injected the baby with monoclonal antibodies primed to bind
with the invading T cells to halt the potentially fatal reaction.

At the Dana-Farber Cancer Institute in Boston, researchers used
monoclonal antibodies to cure a child suffering from severe com-

bined *immune deficiency* (SCID), a disorder similar to AIDS except that it is present at birth. The researchers treated with monoclonal antibodies a bone marrow transplant from the baby's mother and also gave monoclonals to the child. Six weeks after the transplant, the grafted marrow began to produce T cells compatible with the child's tissues.

The Dana-Farber researchers are using a combination of monoclonals and standard therapy to treat leukemia patients, mostly children. Drugs and radiation are used to eliminate the visible leukemia cells; marrow is treated with monoclonal antibodies to destroy remaining cancer cells and then returned to the body.

At Johns Hopkins University in Baltimore, Dr. Stanley Order has chemically bonded radioactive iodine to monoclonal antibodies to treat patients with liver cancer. There have been remissions and shrunken tumors.

At the Texas Health Science Center in Dallas, ricin, a deadly extract of the castor bean, has been bonded to monoclonals and tested for use in leukemic cells in the bone marrow of mice. The tumor cells have been destroyed and normal cells saved. In another experiment, cancers went into remission when mice were treated with radiation to eliminate 90 percent of the cancers and monoclonals were used to kill the rest of the cancerous cells.

At the University of Texas Health Center in San Antonio, a monoclonal antibody has been developed to identify and monitor a bladder-cancer marker in urine. It accurately identified 83 percent of the urine specimens for cancer.

Researchers at several cancer centers are investigating the use of monoclonal antibodies for detecting cancer, including melanoma and cancers of the colon, breast, and ovary. These special radioactive antibodies seek out cancer cells and attach themselves only to those kinds of cells. The radioactive "hot spots" where the antibodies have lodged can be photographed with X rays. Because antibodies from breast cancer can be sent to search out breast cancer, and colon tumor antibodies can search out colon tumors, it is hoped that this technique can possibly be used to find specific cancers earlier.

Are all monoclonal antibodies in the testing stage, or are some being used commercially?
There already are some commercial uses for monoclonal antibodies. For instance, they are being used for early pregnancy testing and for diagnosing various viral diseases. A pellet coated with an antibody will change color when the antibody attaches to the proteins in a sample of urine or blood.

Can monoclonal antibodies be used to kill cancer cells?
Four ways that monoclonal antibodies may be used to kill cancer cells are being studied. They are as follows:

1. Injecting them into the patient's bloodstream and letting them work on their own to search out and destroy cancer cells.
2. Adding a protein (called a complement) to them before they are injected to strengthen their ability to destroy the cancer cells.
3. Attaching chemotherapy drugs to them before they are injected; when they find the cancer cells, the drug would be released, destroying the cancer cells and not the normal tissue.
4. Attaching radioactive isotopes to the antibodies, which would deliver radiation directly to the cancer cells.

Thymosin

What is thymosin?
Thymosin is a hormone produced by the thymus. The parent hormone of interferon, it was first isolated from the thymus gland in 1965 and is already proving to be of value in treating children born without normal immunity. Experimental and clinical studies are presently being conducted in more than 100 research centers in the United States and Europe to test thymosin's effectiveness in animals and also in people with infectious diseases, cancer, and other diseases associated with the immune system. Dr. Allan L. Goldstein and his colleagues at the George Washington University Medical Center in Washington, D.C., developed the method for accurately measuring the amount of thymosin in the blood. They have found that there are very high levels of the hormone in newborn children and that it declines significantly with age and with specific diseases.

What sort of research is being done with thymosin?

There are several hundred research projects around the world involving thymosin. Researchers at George Washington University Medical Center, Washington, D.C., say they are already able to use it to reverse the immunosuppressive effects of steroids (such as are used to treat severe rheumatoid arthritis) and of chemotherapy being used in cancer treatment. One of the major applications is combining thymosin with radiation therapy for some lung cancers. Trials with thymosin are being conducted on patients with multiple sclerosis, lupus, and rheumatoid arthritis. It is also being used on patients who are at risk for AIDS, as well as on AIDS patients themselves to help ward off opportunistic infections.

What specific tests are being performed with thymosin?

Two forms of thymosin are being tested: thymosin fraction 5 (TF_5), which is an extract from calf thymus tissue; and alpha-1, which is synthetically produced. Early results indicate that patients with locally advanced non-small cells lung cancer showed improved T-cell function and improved survival, according to the National Cancer Institute. Further testing in lung cancer is under way.

Thymosin has also meant the difference between life and death for some children born with rare immune-deficiency ailments. It is being tested in patients with disorders now recognized as related to the "T-cell" arm of the immune system.

Interferon

How was interferon discovered?

Interferon was discovered when two scientists at the National Institute of Medical Research in London, Dr. Alick Isaacs and Dr. Jean Lindemann, were trying to solve the mystery of why cells that were infected by a virus became resistant to other viruses. They found that cells from chick embryos which were infected with influenza gave out a substance that, when added to other cells, made those cells resistant to virus. The substance was named interferon because it was able to "interfere" with virus infection.

Are there different kinds of interferon?

Yes. Interferon, an impure protein produced by the white cells as the first line of defense against viral infection, is normally manufactured by cells in response to chemical stimuli. Interferon triggers a chemical reaction that protects healthy cells, while stimulating killer cells in the body's immune system to attack infected cells.

Interferons are divided into three classes: alpha, beta, and gamma. They are further divided according to the cell type from which the interferon comes: leukocytes (white blood cells), lymphoblasts (precursors of immune cells), and fibroblasts (connective-tissue cells). In addition, scientists classify interferons based on which are produced naturally by the body and which are produced synthetically by inserting interferon genes into bacteria to raise a large quantity of the substance.

Researchers originally believed there was only one interferon. They have found, however, that there are many different interferon genes, each with a specific job. Although the interferons are different from each other, they all work together in ways that scientists are still sorting out.

Characteristics of Various Interferons

Type of Interferon	Characteristics	
	Source	Activity
Natural (produced by body)		
Alpha Leukocyte Lymphoblastoid*	Leukocytes and lymphoblasts are stimulated to produce interferon after viral induction.	Antiviral, anticancer. Alters cell surfaces—e.g., by increasing number of antigens on cell surface. Modulation of immune system by stimulation of natural killer lymphocytes and macrophages, and suppression of proliferative responses.
Beta Fibroblast	Fibroblasts are stimulated to produce interferon after double-stranded RNA induction.	Same as for alpha interferons.

*Beta is removed from purified product given to patients.

| TYPE OF INTERFERON | CHARACTERISTICS | |
	Source	*Activity*
Gamma Immune	White blood cells are stimulated to produce this interferon after mitogen or antigen stimulation.	Anticancer activity in various cancer cell lines different from that seen with alpha or beta interferons. *In vitro*, gamma interferon has more potent macrophage-stimulating activity and less potent NK-augmenting activity than alpha IFN.
Synthetically Produced Alpha Leukocyte Lymphoblastoid	*E. coli* bacteria, containing nucleic acids derived from human leukocytes. Not available.	Similar to leukocyte interferon extracted from human cells.
Beta Fibroblast	*E. coli* bacteria, containing nucleic acids derived from human fibroblasts.	Highly purified preparation with biological activity *in vitro*.
Gamma Immune	*E. coli* bacteria, containing nucleic acids derived from human leukocytes.	Antiviral activity. Antitumor activity not yet determined.

Against what diseases are interferons effective?

There are some viral diseases that have responded to interferon, including hepatitis, some respiratory viruses, warts, herpes simplex, and shingles. People who are treated with interferon seem to have shorter and less severe sicknesses. It is still too early to tell how effective interferon is; it may be 5 to 10 years before all the evidence is in.

Is interferon effective in treating cancer?

In animals trial, interferon has been most effective when it has been given at the same time or shortly after an animal has been inoculated with a tumor. Large tumors have not responded well to interferon. It is thought that interferon may not directly kill cancer cells, as do the conventional drugs, but may slow their rate of growth and division so that they become sluggish and die. Interferon also seems to be a better anticancer drug when combined with a chemotherapy drug. Phase II trials (where the antitumor activity of the drug is determined in several specific cancers) have shown at least a 50 percent decrease in tumor size in occasional patients with breast cancer, melanoma, and a few miscellaneous solid tumors. Response rates in patients with kidney-cell cancer appear to be higher. More than half of the lymphoma patients have responded to alpha interferon, and very high response rates (over 50 percent) have been seen in hairy-cell leukemia and chronic granulocytic leukemia. Interferon also seems to be working against Kaposi's sarcoma, the cancer associated with AIDS, and against multiple myeloma, cancer of the bone marrow cells. There are dozens of investigational trials under way using different kinds of interferons for various cancers.

Tumor Necrosis Factor

What is tumor necrosis factor?

The existence of tumor necrosis factor was suspected based on an observation made many years ago by doctors that occasionally a cancer patient would improve after a bout with a serious infection. Scientists have speculated that when the immune system responds to an infection it also produces a substance that destroys tumor cells. Tumor necrosis factor occurs naturally in very small amounts in humans and other animals. Researchers have succeeded in cloning tumor necrosis factor, or TNF, which seems to be the magic substance.

Laboratory tests in animals show that animals with cancer have lost the ability to produce tumor necrosis factor in their own bodies. Research conducted in Japan found that TNF, produced artificially by genetic engineering techniques from a human gene, can selectively destroy malignant cells, in many forms of cancer, when applied in the laboratory on cancer cells. Normal cells are virtually not affected. In addition, gamma interferon seems to show more activity against cancer when combined with TNF, with the interferon suppressing tumor-cell growth while the TNF destroys the tumors already there. Human trials with tumor necrosis factor are just beginning.

What is colony-stimulating factor-1?

Colony-stimulating factor-1 is a protein that stimulates the body's production of macrophages, white blood cells that act as scavengers. One of several proteins that the body produces naturally in extremely small amounts to govern the growth and development of the immune system's white blood cells, colony-stimulating factor-1 helps activate the macrophages to attack foreign invaders.

Researchers have cloned the gene and used it to induce animal cells to produce samples of the pure substance. They hope to engineer bacteria or yeasts to produce the material for future laboratory experiments. It is anticipated that it can be used in humans to augment the resistance to infections provided by a person's own macrophages. Tests in animals are presently under way.

What is interleukin-2?

Interleukin-2, called IL-2 for short, is a substance used to activate immune system cells in fighting cancer. Scientists at the National Cancer Institute have been using IL-2 to treat patients with advanced cancers who had failed to respond to any other treatment. In the first twenty-five patients treated, one's cancer disappeared completely and the tumors of ten others shrank in size by at least 50 percent.

The treatment removes circulating white blood cells from the patient, mixes them with mass-produced IL-2 to convert them into killer cells, and then reinjects them into the patient's blood with large doses of IL-2. The killer cells in the patient's body multiply and start attacking the tumor. Six medical centers have begun using this treatment for advanced patients with melanoma, colon, and kidney cancers: New England Cancer Center, Boston; Montefiore Medical Center, Bronx, New York; University of

Texas Health Science Center, San Antonio; Cancer Research Institute of the Medical Center at the University of California, San Francisco; Loyola University Medical Center, Maywood, Illinois; and City of Hope National Medical Center, Duarte, California. M.D. Anderson Hospital and Tumor Institute, Houston, Texas, and Wisconsin Clinical Center, Madison, are also treating patients with IL-2.

Organ Transplants

Why does the body reject a transplanted organ?
The body recognizes the new organ as a foreign invader and launches a fierce immunologic attack aimed at destroying the donated tissues much as it fights off dangerous microorganisms. Rejection is an ever-present threat with any transplant and is an almost inevitable complication of heart transplants, occurring in 90 percent of transplant recipients. The rejection can strike unpredictably, with episodes lasting from a few hours to days. Episodes can recur at any time, alternating with long periods when the body tolerates the donated organ well. One of the mysteries is why rejections strike at a particular time and why they tend to diminish the longer the organ is in place. Scientists are trying to develop new tools to help diagnose rejection in its earliest stages. They believe that repeated, prolonged episodes of rejection can be more dangerous than a single episode, and they are working on methods to minimize the number of rejection episodes.

Why doesn't the mother's body reject a fetus?
This question has been puzzling scientists for decades. Since half of the placenta's genetic makeup comes from the father, the placenta is, in effect, a graft. Yet the mother's system does not reject the placenta as it would a transplanted lung or kidney. Many biochemicals taken from the urine of pregnant women have been tested as the possible immunosuppressive that could inhibit the mother's rejection response. One, named *uromodulin* by the researchers from the National Cancer Institute who isolated it, may play a role in preventing rejection of the placenta and fetus. The scientists have found that when certain white cells are isolated and grown in culture, uromodulin inhibits their activity when added at the beginning of the culture. This suggests that it interferes with an early stage of the immune response. If this theory holds up under further inspection, uromodulin could join the growing list of newly discovered immune system modulators,

such as interleukin-1 and -2, interferon, and tumor necrosis factor.

1949–1950: Sir Peter Medawar found that mice could be made to accept skin grafts from other mice if the fetus was injected with donor cells.

What is chronic rejection?
Patients who survive the initial threats of having the body reject a transplanted organ can develop another complication, called chronic rejection, in which rejection reactions recur. These usually occur within 3 months after the transplant operation. Chronic rejection is an accelerated form of arteriosclerosis, affecting the blood vessels transversing the heart as well as the coronary arteries. If the patient develops chronic rejection, the physician will consider giving the patient another transplant.

How long must transplant patients continue taking antirejection drugs?
Except for identical twins, people who have had organ transplants must continue to take antirejection drugs for the rest of their lives.

Researchers at the Ontario Cancer Institute in Toronto have conducted conditioning experiments with mice by giving them skin grafts from genetically different mice, which produced a strong response from the immune system to reject the transplant. The mice then had surgical casts placed around their abdomens. After several operations the mice were given surgical casts, although no grafts were performed. Blood tests showed that the level of lymphocyte precursors (cells that mature into lymphocytes) in the mice with casts only was three times as high as normal, exactly the same level that the actual operation produced.

What role do blood transfusions play in organ transplants?
Blood transfusions from organ donors play an important role in preventing the rejection of organ transplants. Researchers are now investigating preoperative transfusions of the donor's blood to desensitize the recipient's body to the new organ. Physicians at the University of Alabama have had some success with taking blood from the donor, storing it for 42 days, and giving the blood to the recipient weekly before the surgery. The stored donor

blood, it is believed, in some way alters the immune system to reduce the possibility of rejection.

What are human leukocyte antigens?

*H*uman *l*eukocyte *a*ntigens (HLA) are the markers on the surface of white blood cells that are used to match compatible recipients with donors for the transplantation of kidneys, hearts, or other organs. There are more than eighty different marker substances that must be taken into consideration in determining HLA tissue types. This is why it is so difficult to find a close match in planning an organ transplant. Compare HLA matching with blood typing, where only four antigen markers—labeled A, B, O, and Rh—determine blood compatibility. It is apparent that the HLA substances are crucial to the regulation of the body's natural immune defense system.

What sorts of diseases can be detected by HLA markers?

Many of the diseases linked to the HLA system are believed to be somehow related to the autoimmune processes in which the body's defense system attacks some of the body's own tissues. Rheumatoid arthritis, systemic lupus, juvenile diabetes, and myasthenia gravis are just a few of the diseases in which particular HLA types are most commonly found.

How can HLA be used to advantage in the future?

By identifying the specific characteristic HLA markers that signal specific diseases, scientists feel that they will, in the future, be able to warn a person when he or she is at particular risk of acquiring a certain disease. Sometimes such early warning by itself will allow the person to change lifestyle patterns and thereby avoid the disease.

What is cyclosporin-A?

Cyclosporin-A is a soil-fungus derivative with potent immunosuppressive properties, used to improve the success rate of transplants. Cyclosporin-A has been used on patients with kidney, liver, or heart transplants to suppress the natural immune response so that the new organ can be tolerated. It appears to block the T-helper lymphocytes, the white blood cells believed to play a key role in attacking transplanted organs. Cyclosporin-A also does not severely depress functioning in the bone marrow, where many of the white blood cells needed to fight infections are formed. The use of this substance also allows the reduction of steroid drug dosage and seems to reduce severity of rejection attacks.

Is cyclosporine being tested for use in immune diseases?

Dr. Robert Handschumacher and colleagues at the Yale Comprehensive Cancer Center, New Haven, Connecticut, doing research involving cyclosporine, have found high levels of receptors for the substance on T cells. They have isolated the receptor, named it cyclophilin and determined its structure. They have found the same receptor in many body tissues and in other forms of life, including sponges and some parasites. They theorize that since it is found in so many tissues, it may be a regulator of the entire system. They also believe that when cyclosporine covers the receptor, it may prevent a natural substance made by the body from regulating the immune system. The existence of the receptors indicates there is such a substance, and when the immune response is weakened in various illnesses, they think it may be because there is too much of this immune suppressant in the body. Thirty percent of patients with lupus have antibodies against this receptor, and it is found in high levels in colon cancer tissue.

Is cyclosporine being used to treat cancer?

The Yale researchers are using cyclosporine in treating T-cell leukemia, where T cells multiply wildly, do not perform normally, and crowd out other blood cells. It does not kill T cells but suppresses their function temporarily.

Bone Marrow Transplants

What is a bone marrow transplant?

A bone marrow transplant replaces a patient's abnormal or diseased marrow with healthy marrow from a donor. The ideal donor is an identical twin. However, there is a 25 percent chance that any one brother or sister will have the same proteins (HLA antigen) as the patient, since these proteins are inherited from the parents—one set from the mother and one from the father.

Many Americans remember the poignant, much-publicized case of David, who, because his immune system was not functioning (he had SCID), lived all his life in a bubble that provided a germ-free environment. Many also remember the decision by his doctors to attempt to free him from the plastic bubble. A bone marrow transplant was performed, using marrow from his 15-year-old sister, in hopes of giving him a chance for a normal life. Unfortunately, the transplant was unsuccessful. After David's death, the autopsy confirmed that a common virus, Epstein-Barr, which is carried by more than 90 percent of the population, was responsible for the failure of the procedure. The virus took up residence in the few B lymphoctyes David had and began to grow wildly. David's near-total lack of T cells allowed the growth to continue unchecked. Then cancer, a B-cell lymphoma, developed. Researchers believe that David's case established proof that there is a link between the common Epstein-Barr virus and the growth of the cancer. Doctors speculate that if the bone marrow transplant had been successful, David might have developed immune agents in time to fight off the Epstein-Barr virus.

Why are bone marrow transplants performed?
A bone marrow transplant may be performed to help the body to produce normal marrow cells or to replace normal ones that have been destroyed along with tumor cells during chemotherapy or radiation therapy.

What is graft-versus-host disease?
This condition occurs with bone marrow transplants in which cells produced by donated marrow attack the patient's own tissues.

Are there new methods being used for bone marrow transplants?
Many transplant teams around the world are investigating new techniques. They include using an unrelated donor, using specially prepared monoclonal antibodies, and using the patient's own bone marrow by first cleaning the removed bone marrow with monoclonal antibodies or anticancer drugs. The possibility of establishing a donor bank to collect marrow samples from donors in the general population is also being examined. These methods will help to solve some of the problems that have made bone marrow transplants unsuccessful in the past, especially the susceptibility to infection due to the fact that the immune system is not fully reconstituted for as long as 18 months following a transplant.

Are bone marrow transplants being used in infants born with severe combined immune deficiency disease (SCID)?
Yes. Babies born with this disease today are given bone marrow transplants shortly after birth. Dozens of SCID babies have survived the transplants and developed immune systems even when no perfectly matched donor could be found.

ny individuals in a region at the same time, it is consid-
be an epidemic.

chapter 5

Understanding Bacteria and Viruses

History records that infectious diseases and plagues have been with humankind through the ages. It was not until the late 1800s that investigators were able to identify twenty-one microorganisms as specific causes of human diseases. Among these microorganisms were the bacilli that cause typhoid fever, tuberculosis, and diphtheria; the pneumococcus and the meningococcus, responsible for the commonest forms of pneumonia and meningitis; and the streptococcus, which is responsible for scarlet fever, septic sore throat, and childbed fever as well as for infections in other organs and the bloodstream. Because of incomplete knowledge, bacteriological discoveries did little to help victims of the infectious diseases. It was not until later that true progress was made in learning to prevent the spread of disease.

As knowledge and awareness began to grow, scientists, using ever-more-potent microscopes, have piled discovery upon discovery to help wipe out many of the infectious diseases that had always been presumed to be an inevitable part of life. Our bodies are still vulnerable to the same disease-causing bacteria, viruses, fungi, and parasites that abound in our atmosphere. What has changed is the understanding we have of how viruses and bacteria grow, how vaccines can prevent them from overrunning our bodies, and how they can be successfully treated. The growing science of immunology is shedding new light on how the immune system deals with bacteria and viruses.

What is an epidemic?
Usually, when a contagious disease breaks out suddenly and af-

fects many individuals in a region at the same time, it is considered to be an epidemic.

What is pandemic disease?

A pandemic disease is a widespread epidemic, one that breaks out in many areas at the same time—throughout several regions, across a continent, or globally.

What are the two types of infectious agents?

One class of infectious agents consists of single-cell organisms including bacteria, protozoa, fungi, and rickettsiae. The other class contains viruses, which are actually much simpler organisms than bacteria. However, because of the way they cause infection, they are more difficult to destroy.

What are some rickettsial diseases?

Rickettsial diseases include Rocky Mountain spotted fever, which is spread through ticks, and typhus, which is transmitted to humans by lice. Rickettsiae are microbes that, like bacteria, have cell walls and require oxygen but, like viruses, depend on living cells for growth. The rickettsiae are usually carried by insects. Once they enter the body, they multiply in the cells of small blood vessels.

What kinds of diseases are caused by fungal infections?

Fungal infections include such diseases as candidiasis, which is responsible for vaginal infections and thrush; ringworm, a fungal skin disease characterized by ring-shaped lesions on the body; and athlete's foot, which causes scaling and blisters between the toes. Fungi include molds, mildews, yeasts, and some one-celled microbes.

Bacteria

What are bacteria?

Bacteria are one-celled microorganisms that play many roles in the body, ranging from harmless to beneficial and from virulent to lethal. "Friendly" kinds of bacteria, for example, live on our skins, leaving no foothold for less desirable invaders, as the compounds they produce inhibit other microorganisms. The mucus in our throats is an effective trap for harmful bacteria. In the windpipe, ciliated cells push mucus containing inhaled dust particles and bacteria toward the throat so that they can be coughed out or swallowed. If swallowed, the bacteria pass down the esophagus to be destroyed by the hydrochloric acid in the stomach.

Disease-causing bacteria are single-cell microbes that carry on relatively complex metabolic functions. They can reproduce within the body, destroying healthy tissues, and release toxic substances. One way bacteria succeed in entering the body and causing infection is when tissue is damaged by chemicals or by physical force. If bacteria seize such an opportunity to invade the tissue, they may multiply in great numbers and cause infection. Within a few hours, however, circulating white blood cells are attracted to the site of the infection and begin to engulf the bacteria and any dead or damaged cells.

What are antibiotics?

Antibiotics are a large class of substances produced by a variety of microorganisms and fungi. They have the power to arrest the growth of or destroy bacteria. Antibiotics destroy cells in a number of ways: by punching holes in them; by interfering with the cell's ability to stabilize new cell surface product; or by entering the cells and disrupting the mechanisms used in synthesizing DNA, RNA, and proteins.

Antibiotics save the lives of thousands of people each year. However, each time a person takes antibiotics, some of the friendly bacteria in the body are destroyed, providing an opportunity for harmful bacteria to flourish. Antibiotics are effective with diseases that are caused by bacteria—such as strep throat, bacterial pneumonia, and meningitis. They are useless, however, in treating viruses.

How do antibiotics work?

Antibiotics combat bacterial infections by interfering with the essential life processes of the bacteria. Penicillin, for example, prevents the production of bacterial cell membranes, the protective cell wall without which bacteria cannot exist.

Do antibiotics kill both protective and harmful bacteria?

It is true that antibiotics often kill the protective strains of bacteria that normally help the body to resist infections. Some physicians recommend that patients taking antibiotics eat a small amount of yogurt with active cultures daily to help offset the effect of antibiotics on protective bacteria.

Why aren't antibiotics used against viruses?

Antibiotics generally are not effective against viral diseases, although they may be prescribed to prevent bacterial infections that sometimes accompany these diseases.

Viruses

What are viruses?
Unlike bacteria, which are free-living organisms, viruses are essentially parasitic, dependent upon living cellular material for their survival. They are more difficult to study than bacteria because live animals, fertilized eggs, or tissue cultures are required for laboratory observation of viral activity. Normally, in a process called replication, a virus attaches itself to the host cell at predetermined receptor sites, then penetrates the cell and loses its outer coat, releasing nuclear material—DNA or RNA—which is then reassembled and released by the cell. It is now infectious, and vulnerable to the host's defense mechanisms.

What are the two major types of viruses?
There are two major types of viruses, those with genetic material consisting only of DNA and those with only RNA. Most virus-related cancers in humans have been linked to DNA viruses, although some recent studies have also uncovered evidence linking RNA viruses to some forms of human cancers.

Do viruses affect plants and animals as well as people?
Yes. Not only do they attack plants, animals, and people, but even bacteria are not spared from attack by viruses. The agents that attack bacteria are called bacteriophages.

How big are viruses?
It was not until the advent of electron microscopy in the 1950s that anyone was able to see a virus. A single virus is about 1/100th the size of a bacterium—so small that about 10,000 can fit on the head of a pin.

How do bacterial diseases differ from viral diseases?
Bacteria are one-celled microorganisms that reproduce outside the cell. Viruses, on the other hand, are more complex. They invade a healthy cell, then restructure the machinery within the cell so that the original cell breaks down completely, releasing thousands of newly designed cells that replicate the virus and then attack other cells, thereby spreading disease.

Why are viruses so hard to treat?
Viruses lodge themselves within the host cells. Therefore, treating them means risking injury or death to the cell and is thus very difficult. Since viruses operate slowly, causing illness days

or weeks after entering the body, any effort to combat them after trouble occurs is usually too late.

What are antiviral drugs?

Antiviral drugs are designed to manage an infection by not allowing the virus to grow. Unlike antibiotics, which do their job by killing the single-celled bacteria that float around the bloodstream and cause infection, antiviral drugs inhibit the viral replication process. If administered soon enough, an antiviral drug can keep an infection under control. There are now a number of antiviral drugs approved for prescription use in the United States.

What kinds of drugs are being studied for antiviral uses?

The interferons, normally produced in the body, are one group of drugs that shows great promise for combating viral diseases. Although interferons were originally hailed as a possible magic bullet for cancer treatment, further study indicates that they have great potential for future usefulness in preventing the common cold—though the nasal irritation caused by the drug continues to be a problem. Ribavirin, another experimental antiviral, is believed to be useful in the more than 10 percent of lower-respiratory-tract infections that are characterized by hacking coughs, high fever, and weakness. There are indications that this compound can shorten the duration of influenza attacks, and can combat a variety of viruses. This drug allows the virus to replicate in the cells but causes the copies to be faulty and incapable of surviving to spread infection. Most major pharmaceutical companies are working on antiviral programs, and clinical trials of a number of experimental compounds are under way.

Do some viruses reside in the body permanently?

It appears that some do. The viruses that cause warts and infectious hepatitis remain in the body after the initial attack and may be activated again and again. *Herpes zoster,* the virus that causes chicken pox, can be reactivated much later in life to cause painful shingles. Cold sores, caused by the *herpes simplex* virus, appear again and again.

What are slow viruses?

They are called slow viruses because they appear to be responsible for prolonged infection and gradual degeneration of the nervous system, incubating for years—even decades—before they attack the brain or nervous system. It is believed by some that there may be a slow-virus link to rheumatoid arthritis, multiple sclerosis, and Alzheimer's disease. These slow-virus diseases are sometimes referred to as unconventional virus diseases because scientists suspect that they may be caused by a class of viruslike agents unlike other known viruses.

What are retroviruses?

Retroviruses are viruses that have been recognized since the early 1900s as causes of cancers in chickens and other animals. They have been studied by researchers because of the clues they offer to the nature of cancer and even to the basic organization of life. Retroviruses appear to have the ability to be used as vehicles for transplanting genes from one species to another. Their complete roles are still not fully understood.

In 1980, Dr. Robert C. Gallo and his group of researchers at the National Cancer Institute linked some leukemia and lymphoma patients with what appeared to be a retrovirus. Subsequently the virus has been found in many areas of the world, including the United States, the Caribbean region, and Africa. Known as HTLV-I, the retrovirus is generally regarded as the first cancer-causing human retrovirus. A closely related virus called HTLV-II has recently been found in one cancer patient and in one chronic drug abuser, but has not been linked with certainty to human disease. These retrovirus cells, though they do not have oncogenes, have been cloned and analyzed and can transform cells growing in the laboratory into a cancerlike state. A third member of the family of retroviruses, known as HTLV-III, is considered to be the cause of AIDS. A virus linked to AIDS discovered by scientists in France and named LAV is now generally believed to be identical to HTLV-III. More recent research has found evidence of something resembling a retrovirus in a puzzling category of hepatitis infections. The link to hepatitis still remains to be confirmed.

Since viruses are known to be contagious, and some viruses may cause cancer, does that then mean that some cancers are contagious?

Actually, the viral infections that increase the risk of cancer may be contagious, but the cancer itself is not. What has been demonstrated is that there may be a greater risk of cancer following virus infections; however, only a small fraction of those infected will develop cancer as a result of the virus. Again, some immune systems seem to be more capable than others in preventing the onset of the second stage of the disease.

How do scientists test viruses to determine if they have links with cancer?

Scientists use the following set of standards for the kinds of evidence necessary to link a virus and a tumor:

- Presence of antivirus antibody, or of elevated levels of such antibody, more often than in controls, especially before the disease develops
- Presence of viral genome (DNA or RNA) in tissue
- Ability of the virus to transform cells in culture
- Ability of the virus to induce tumors in experimental animals
- Detection of the virus or the viral genome in experimental tumors

The final test would be the demonstration that elimination of the virus reduces the incidence of the disease.

What are prions?

Prions, which take their name from the words *proteinaceous infectious particle*, are much smaller than the smallest viruses. Unlike viruses or bacteria, they appear to contain no genetic material but to consist only of protein. This puzzles scientists, because it complicates the problem of understanding how prions cause disease as well as how they reproduce. Another unusual characteristic of prions is that their presence evokes no detectable response from the immune defense system.

Prions were discovered in 1982 by Dr. Stanley Prusiner, a neurologist at the University of California, San Francisco, and his colleagues. The researchers were studying scrapie, a fatal disease in sheep that afflicts the brain and central nervous system. In January 1985, a report in the *New England Journal of Medicine* identified prions as the cause of Creutzfeldt-Jakob disease, a rare human illness with symptoms similar to those of scrapie. (See p. 179.)

Is there any evidence that viruses weaken the immune system?

The fact that viruses weaken the immune system is firmly established. Microbiologists have a set of criteria, known as Koch's postulates, that are used as a standard to determine if a disease has a viral source. The criteria, established by Koch in 1890, include the following:

- The organism is regularly found in lesions of the disease.
- The organism can be isolated in pure culture on artificial media.
- Inoculation of this culture produces a similar disease in experimental animals.
- The organism can be recovered from the lesions in these experimental animals.

Vaccines

What is a vaccine?

A vaccine is a dose of just enough of a particular bacteria or virus to trigger the immune system but not enough to make the inoculated person sick. The vaccine supplements the body's natural immunity by introducing into the body small quantities of the antigen, enough to stimulate antibody production but not enough to produce disease. Another method of producing vaccine is to use antigens that have been detoxified in some way but whose antigen structure remains unaltered, so they can still trigger an immune response, making the person immune to that particular bacteria or virus.

Do vaccines cure infectious diseases?

Vaccines are designed to *prevent* infectious diseases. They do not cure them.

How and when did the concept of vaccination originate?

The word *vaccine* is derived from the Latin word for cow, *vacca*. In 1796, Edward Jenner, an English doctor, observed that milkmaids who caught cowpox from cows did not catch the deadly smallpox. He tried rubbing pus from the cow's pox into people's skin to somehow protect them from smallpox. We now know that the pus contained the cowpox virus. Since cowpox is a weak relative of the smallpox virus, the cowpox antibodies produced in the bodies of infected individuals helped to immunize them against smallpox.

Many physicians in England were adamantly opposed to the practice of vaccination. They reasoned that the cowpox vaccine would produce cowlike faces, cause cow hair to grow on women, and cause men to bellow like bulls. That was in 1798, but subsequent events proved the value of Jenner's findings—and vaccination has succeeded in almost banishing the once feared and fatal scourge of smallpox from the face of the earth.

The entire technology on which today's vaccines are based actually stems from Jenner's theory of using related germs or altered germs to fight more powerful viruses and bacteria. Because many germs do not have relationships as close as that between smallpox and cowpox, scientists experimented with weakening strong viruses in the laboratory.

On a tombstone in Dorset, England, is the following inscription:

To the Memory of Benjamin Jesty who departed this life April 16th, 1816, aged 79 Years. He was born at Yetminster in this County, and was an upright honest Man: particularly noted for having been the first Person (known) that introduced the Cow Pox by Inoculation, and who from his great strength of mind made the Experiment from the Cow on his Wife and two Sons in the Year 1774.

The adjoining gravestone attests to the fact that his wife survived the vaccination, having died in 1824, aged 84.

How do scientists develop vaccines?
They use all or part of a particular germ against which they are seeking protection. First they weaken, dismember, or kill the germ in the laboratory. When injected into the human body as a vaccine, the weakened germ triggers the body to produce the antigen-specific proteins called antibodies. These antibodies keep the deadly germs from reproducing in the body.

What is a killed-virus vaccine?
A killed-virus vaccine contains viruses that have been killed by chemical treatment. Killed-virus vaccines carry no danger of the recipient acquiring infection from the vaccine, but booster shots are required periodically.

What is a live-virus vaccine?
Live-virus vaccines are made using a strain of virus that has been weakened by careful breeding in the laboratory; the microbes,

however, are still alive. Though live-virus vaccines confer longer-lasting immunity than killed-virus vaccines, there is a slight danger that the vaccine can cause the illness if the treated vaccine reverts to the virulent type.

Are vaccines completely safe?

While it is true that vaccines made from both live and killed viruses carry a small amount of risk, the benefits outweigh the risks. There is controversy in the medical field over the relative safety of live versus killed viruses and bacteria. Those in favor of live vaccines point to the success of the live Sabin polio vaccine, which practically wiped out polio. However, though it is considered one of the safest vaccines, the Sabin vaccine causes five to ten cases of polio each year in the United States. Though it protects the person who receives the vaccine from the disease, the virus can, in rare instances, remain strong enough to infect.

Is there any danger in giving children vaccination shots?

There can be a slight risk. For instance, the pertussis (whooping cough) component of the DPT (*d*iphtheria, *p*ertussis, *t*etanus) vaccine causes severe reactions in a tiny fraction of the children who are vaccinated, estimated to be one case in 310,000 doses. These reactions can include seizures, brain damage, and even death. High-risk children can be those with a family history of seizures, neurological problems, or severe allergies. If you have a family history of any of these problems or if your child or other children in your family have had any reactions to the vaccine or to previous shots, be sure to discuss the problem with your doctor before your child is vaccinated.

What are the different ways in which scientists are using technology to produce new vaccines?

They are growing viruses and bacteria in test tubes to produce the raw material for vaccines. They have learned to alter the genes of viruses and bacteria so that they stimulate the body to produce more antibodies without producing disease. And they are isolating pieces of germs that can trigger immunity against the whole germ.

What kinds of vaccines will we be seeing in the future?

Vaccines made through gene-splicing methods are already appearing on the market. Experimental vaccines have been made against herpes and hepatitis virus, using the method known as gene transfer, where a gene from the virus is isolated and transferred into a harmless virus. To the body, this virus looks and behaves enough like the infectious virus to stimulate the production of antibodies.

against herpes and hepatitis virus using the method known as gene transfer, where a gene from the virus is notted and then

chapter 6

When Immunity Fails and Viruses Attack

Viruses, those troublesome parasitic organisms, were never even seen before the 1950s, when the electron microscope was invented. One hundred times smaller than bacteria, these organisms hide within the cells and are the cause of many diseases, from the common cold to AIDS to a rare disease of New Guinea natives known as kuru. Some viruses live permanently in the body, causing recurring cases of warts or infectious hepatitis long after the initial attack.

The agent or agents responsible for many of our most virulent contagions remain a mystery. Simply identifying the causal agent is only half the battle anyway. The virus that causes polio had been identified long before a vaccine to prevent the disease was finally produced. Flu viruses have been isolated and vaccines developed to combat them, but a slightly altered virus can cause new epidemics to spread unchecked. Finding the key to any of the diseases for which there are still no answers—AIDS, multiple sclerosis, Creutzfeldt-Jakob disease—will unlock many secrets of the immunological process itself.

Colds

What is the definition of a cold?
A cold is a viral infection of the linings of the upper respiratory tract. Specific viruses enter and eventually kill the cells in the mucous membranes of the nose and throat. The cold symptoms that we experience are the result of the body's immune system reactions to the viral invasion. The remedies we usually use to

"treat" a cold alleviate the symptoms but do nothing to combat the viral infection. In fact, *they probably interfere with the body's natural defense.* The membranes in the nose and throat produce mucus that traps inhaled dust, pollen, bacteria, and viruses. The cilia, millions of tiny hairlike projections, move in unison to propel the mucus back through the nose and up the windpipe to the esophagus. Once in the digestive tract, the mucus is swallowed and the infectious agents are eventually destroyed.

What viruses are responsible for the common cold?

It appears that rhinoviruses cause about 25 percent of common colds—primarily those that occur in fall and winter. Coronoviruses cause about 8 percent of colds, mostly those that occur in winter and spring. An additional 10 percent of all colds are caused by influenza and parainfluenza viruses. About half of all common colds are caused by other viruses.

How does the cold virus operate?

The cold virus penetrates the protective blanket of mucus in the nose and throat and attacks the living cells underneath. The protein coat around the virus's genetic material attaches itself to the cells of the mucous membrane. The virus then injects its genetic material into the cell and compels the cell to stop its normal function and turn its resources to making more viruses. As many as a thousand new viruses may come bursting out of a single cell. The new viruses attack surrounding cells and the process continues.

How does the infected cell react to the cold virus?

When the new viruses come bursting from the original cell, the infected cell releases a substance called interferon into the intercellular fluid. This alerts neighboring healthy cells to the invasion and triggers them to produce antiviral chemicals.

What causes all the discomfort of a cold?

The discomfort of a cold results from the body's attempts to cure itself. Membrane cells begin to release substances such as histamine into the intercellular space. Histamine causes dilation of the blood capillaries. Then all the symptoms we normally associate with a cold begin to come into play. More blood flows through the expanded blood vessels, so the affected area reddens. Blood plasma, along with some important defensive chemicals, seeps through the stretched walls of the blood vessels, causing the tissue of the mucous membrane to swell. This narrows the nasal passages and produces congestion. The narrowing of the nasal passages means that not all the mucus can be disposed of through the nose passages, and so the nose starts to run. Nerve endings in the nose sense the swelling and cell destruction, and so the brain responds by forcing a sneeze. Nerves sense an overabundance of mucus—more than the cilia can carry up to the esophagus—and a cough clears the passage before the mucus can descend to the lungs.

What causes a sore throat?
If there has been a viral invasion of the throat, soreness is often accompanied by swollen glands—lymph nodes that have become enlarged because they are trapping the virus and fighting off infection. The throat may also become dry and irritated because of coughing or because of mouth breathing due to a stuffy nose.

What is rhinitis?
Rhinitis is a term used to describe an inflammation of the nose. It usually starts like an ordinary head cold, but it seems to hang on—and becomes a year-round problem. The nose drips, and the head may feel clogged. Sneezing attacks—more than five sneezes at a time, explosive and noisy—are usually symptoms of rhinitis. Often nasal polyps form as a result of nose linings being permanently inflamed.

Does extended isolation increase susceptibility to colds?
In the course of extensive testing done by the Common Cold Unit of Harvard Hospital in Salisbury, England, volunteers were marooned on an island for an entire summer to see if isolation changed their susceptibility to cold viruses. It was found that there did not seem to be any relationship between isolation and susceptibility.

Have researchers tested whether wet feet or wet chilling bring on colds?
This sort of testing has been done at the Common Cold Unit of Harvard Hospital in Salisbury, England, as well as at other research centers. Researchers found little or no connection between this sort of wet chilling and the catching of colds.

What unusual cures for the common cold have been prescribed in the course of human history?
Hippocrates wrote that bleeding was a frequent treatment for a

cold, and Pliny the Elder prescribed "kissing the hairy muzzle of a mouse." The Chinese suggest wrapping a cube of ice to the bottom of each big toe with strips of rag. They leave the ice in place for about 20 minutes. It is recommended that the treatment be repeated several times a day. According to traditional theory, the ice acts to brake the flow of bioenergy past an important cold and influenza control center.

Recent studies have shown that chicken soup, prescribed by Jewish mothers for centuries, seems to be a sensible remedy, since the warm steam clears the nostrils.

Are scientists working on developing a vaccine against colds?
Many scientists feel that with more than 200 infectious agents involved, it would be almost impossible to produce a general cold vaccine, since a vaccine that works against one virus is useless against others. Scientists have recently determined, for the first time, the three-dimensional structure of a common cold virus known as human rhinovirus 14. Using an atom smasher, X-ray images, and a supercomputer, the scientists discovered how parts of the viruses fit together and intertwined; such information is crucial to understanding exactly how the virus manages to infect body cells and how the body's immune system counterattacks and immobilizes the virus. The researchers also noted that the newly discovered structure of the cold virus made prospects for a vaccine to prevent colds seem dim. They had hoped to find a structural feature common to a whole range of cold viruses, but the new discovery did not seem to detect such a feature.

Will the interferon spray prevent colds?
In January 1986, scientists announced what appears to be the first effective drug to prevent symptoms of a rhinovirus infection. The protection against the rhinovirus lasts only as long as the spray is being used, and is not effective in shortening the symptoms of a cold once it appears.

Will the interferon spray work for flu or other viruses?
Scientists were disappointed that the interferon did not protect against influenza virus or other related viruses.

Flu

What does a flu virus look like?
A flu virus looks like a ball studded with spikes. The spikes are two surface proteins called *h*emagglutinin (HA) and *n*euramini-

dase (NA). Inside the virus ball is a thick tangle of genes. Each flu gene is a separate segment of ribonucleic acid (RNA)—eight threads in all. Most other kinds of viruses have a number of different genes fitting onto one strand of nucleic acid. Hemagglutinin is the substance that bashes into a cell during infection and allows the virus access to the cell interior, where it can reproduce. The neuraminidase permits all the viral offspring to break free of the host cell once replication has been completed. Because all of the flu genes are separate units of RNA, they are very flexible. When two different flu viruses happen to infect the same cell, there are suddenly sixteen different genes that can be recombined in different ways for a total of 256 possibilities, creating new hybrids.

> Experiments conducted at the Institute of Experimental Pathology, outside Reykjavík, Iceland, infected seals with a flu virus known as H7N7. This particular virus had been ravaging seal populations along the New England coast, causing serious lung damage. H7N7 is also associated with a lethal form of avian influenza known as fowl plague, which kills chickens in 48 hours by destroying the central nervous system. Robert G. Webster, of St. Jude Children's Research Hospital in Memphis, Tennessee, is regarded as one of the world's leading flu researchers. He tells the story of being a visitor at the Institute of Experimental Pathology when a lab technician was holding a seal infected with the flu virus H7N7. The seal sneezed, spraying the technician. Forty-eight hours after the sneeze incident, the lab technician's eye was red and runny with conjunctivitis. High concentrations of the seal virus were found in the infected eye. Genetic tests determined that the same virus, capable of killing seals in New England and causing eye infections in humans, originated in birds. All eight of the virus genes came from various avian sources.

How dangerous is the flu?

Influenza *annually* kills more people than AIDS has over its entire history. In an age when the flu is viewed by the public as a 3-day nuisance rather than a killer, statistics of past flu epidemics offer a different perspective. Twenty million people died in the

1918–19 pandemic. No one knows why it killed as efficiently as it did, but the 1918 virus felled healthy, able-bodied young people as swiftly as infants and the elderly.

Scientists from St. Jude Children's Research Hospital in Memphis, Tennessee, have been studying the relationship of the duck population to influenza virus since 1974. In the Canadian breeding grounds, they found flu viruses in about 60 to 80 percent of juvenile ducks. All the ducks were healthy. The researchers found viruses floating in lake water and even found different flu viruses cohabiting in the same duck.

Wild ducks harbor every subtype of flu virus, though they seem to be disease free. Flu viruses grow in the cell linings of the intestinal tract, causing no illness, passing easily from duck to duck in pond water. Because ducks migrate great distances, a virus can travel the globe. In genetic studies of the influenza H3N2 virus, which appeared in 1968, there are indications that while seven of its genes came from the previous Asian strain, H2N2, the eighth gene—the one that codes for the all-important hemagglutinin—probably came from a duck. Such an occurrence would have required that someone infected with Asian flu be working with a duck that was also infected—resulting, quite by chance, in a powerful new flu combination.

What does the drug amantadine do?
Amantadine is an important therapeutic tool used to prevent type A flu among high-risk people as well as to thwart the outbreak of epidemics in schools and military bases and to reduce contagion among groups in close contact, such as patients on a hospital ward, or members of a household. It is licensed for use against A strains of influenza, which cause the major pandemic and epidemic outbreaks. Though not fully understood, the drug appears to work by inhibiting the release of infectious viral nucleic acid into the host cell, thereby preventing its spread to other cells. It must be given within 24 hours of the onset of symptoms.

Virus-Related Cancer

Do viruses cause cancer?
Scientists estimate that only about 1 to 5 percent of the cases of

cancer in the United States are related to viruses. However, in some developing countries, the incidence of virus-related cancers is much higher. Even though some so-called "cancer viruses" infect large numbers of people, the number of cancer cases that may be associated with viral infections appears to be very small. It is doubtful that viruses alone are responsible for the development of cancers in humans, because so many people are infected with viruses and relatively few of them ever develop cancer. Therefore, scientists feel that other factors, such as infection with a second virus, the condition of the person's immune or hormonal system, or exposure to substances in the environment may influence a person's susceptibility to virus-linked cancers.

Which human cancers may be caused by viruses?

Human cancers that are virus related are usually linked to the viruses with genetic material consisting only of DNA. Among the DNA viruses, hepatitis B virus, Epstein-Barr virus, herpes simplex II virus, cytomegalovirus, and human papilloma virus have all been linked to cancer in humans. In some populations, chronic infection with hepatitis B virus (hepatitis carriers) increases the risk of developing primary liver cancer (hepatocellular carcinoma) to 223 times the risk for noninfected persons. Hepatitis B vaccine given at a young age in high-risk areas may prevent some liver cancer.

Epstein-Barr virus, the widespread virus that causes infectious mononucleosis in this country, has been strongly linked to Burkitt's lymphoma and nasopharyngeal cancer. Infection with papilloma virus and herpes simplex II virus, in addition to other risk factors, has been associated with the development of cervical cancers.

Recent studies have provided strong evidence that an RNA virus belonging to the class of retroviruses known to cause cancer in animals may cause cancers that affect adult human T cells in the immune system. The virus, called the human T-cell leukemia/lymphoma virus, or HTLV, is the first retrovirus known to cause cancer in humans.

How can a person reduce exposure to the cancer-causing viruses?

Measures to reduce exposure to cancer viruses are most practical against those cancers associated with sexually transmitted viruses such as herpes simplex II, papilloma virus, and cytomegalovirus. These include avoiding multiple sexual partners and using barrier contraceptives. In developing countries, improved sanitary conditions may reduce the spread of Epstein-Barr and hepatitis B virus. Because cancer viruses seldom work alone, elimination of their cofactors, such as insect vectors or hazardous substances in the environment, may reduce spread of the virus.

If cancer is linked to viruses, is it contagious?
No. Viruses associated with cancer may be transmitted from one person to another, but cancer cannot be. Cancer cannot be spread by sneezing, coughing, kissing, or in any other way.

Hepatitis

What are the different kinds of hepatitis?
Type A hepatitis is usually transmitted in food and water contaminated from the urine or stool of an infected person. The virus is excreted in the stool and urine for weeks. Gamma globulin given during the incubation period or prior to traveling in areas where hepatitis is common helps to prevent severe disease.

Type B virus causes serum hepatitis. Usually it is spread by injection or blood transfusion or close contact, such as kissing or sexual intercourse. The type B virus reproduces in amazing quantity in the liver and blood. Symptoms do not appear for 2 to 5 months after exposure, and are similar to those of type A hepatitis—jaundiced skin and eyes, dark urine and light stools.

Hepatitis C, newly discovered, is a retrovirus, a kind of virus that is known to cause only two other diseases in humans: a type of leukemia and *a*quired *i*mmune *d*eficiency *s*yndrome (AIDS). Like hepatitis B, the new version is transmitted through blood and other body fluids. Hepatitis delta virus, another newly described infectious disease, can infect only persons with hepatitis B. A person may be infected with both viruses simultaneously. Superinfection with the delta virus can also occur in someone who is already a hepatitis B carrier. Delta superinfection can transform mild chronic hepatitis B infection to severe progressive active hepatitis and cirrhosis.

How widespread are hepatitis B and C?
It is estimated that about 200,000 new cases of hepatitis B occur each year and that about 800,000 Americans are carriers of the virus. Hepatitis C, the serious and often fatal liver disease, affects as many as 120,000 Americans a year.

Physicians are concerned that cases of hepatitis B could increase, since studies have shown that the hepatitis carrier rate is very high among people now living in this country but who were born in Asia. Since there has been a large influx of Vietnamese and other Asians to this country since 1970—statistics from the Centers for Disease Control show that over 660,000 Asian refugees were resettled in the United States between 1975 and 1983—thousands of babies born of Asian mothers can be at risk of developing liver cancer. The hepatitis B rate has doubled since 1974, partly because of immigration from Asia and partly because of the high rate of the disease among intravenous drug users and male homosexuals. It is spread through sexual intercourse between sexually active male homosexuals as well as by contaminated needles among intravenous drug users.

Where does the hepatitis virus lodge?

The hepatitis virus heads directly for the liver—where it commandeers the cellular genetic and reproductive machinery to create thousands of replicas of itself. These replicas burst forth, killing the host cells, and begin widespread destruction within the body.

Does hepatitis B virus ever turn into cancer?

There is some indication that there is a relationship between hepatitis B and liver cancer (primary hepatocellular carcinoma). Although in the United States and Western Europe liver cancers represent only about 2 percent of all cancers in males and 2.5 percent in females, they are among the most common cancers in other areas of the world—including China, Africa, and the Philippines. These same areas also have a high incidence of hepatitis B. Blood testing of patients in these areas has revealed a significantly greater level of antigens and antibodies of hepatitis B virus than is normal in the Western nations.

A 1981 study in Taiwan involving 19,253 antigen-negative patients and 3454 antigen-positive patients showed that of the 41 men who died of liver cancer during the study, 40 were antigen positive—they had hepatitis B virus—making the risk for the liver cancer 223 to 1 among the men who had been infected with hepatitis B virus. According to the study's authors, this association was "the strongest ever established between a virus and a human neoplasm." Another, smaller study completed in 1982 strengthened these findings by showing that the hepatitis B virus was present in patients' blood years before they developed liver cancer—pointing to the possibility that the infection is a prelude to cancer, rather than secondary to the development of the cancer. There is also an indication that aflatoxin, a toxin produced by mold, and long-term alcohol intake are influential factors in the development of human liver cancers.

> A virus related to hepatitis B virus has been found in wood-chucks belonging to a colony in which 25 percent of the animals die of primary liver cancer.

Can children born to mothers with hepatitis B become carriers of the virus?
It has been found that infants born to mothers with hepatitis B have an 85 percent chance of being infected themselves, becoming lifetime carriers of the virus if not vaccinated shortly after birth. In the past, newborns of mothers with hepatitis B have been given hepatitis B immune globulin, an antibody serum that protects the baby from the disease but does not stimulate a protective response from the infant's immune system. Vaccination can augment the protection provided by the hepatitis B immune globulin, reducing the risk of infection.

Are vaccines available for hepatitis?
A live-virus vaccine against type A hepatitis is being developed. An expensive conventional vaccine, made from a virus protein taken from the donated blood of persons who have been infected with hepatitis B, is available. It is expensive (about $100 for three injections) as well as difficult to make, and it has been avoided by some people because of fear that exposure to a vaccine derived from donated blood might expose them to other blood-born viruses, such as AIDS. Two experimental vaccines, produced through gene-splicing methods, are being tested. Although these vaccines are still in the research stage, it is estimated that one or the other may become generally available in 2 or 3 years. These vaccines will be free from risk of contamination by substances in human blood, will be available in limitless quantities, and will probably be relatively inexpensive. It is estimated that it will probably take about three generations of widespread use to eliminate hepatitis B virus, once the new vaccines become available.

Work is under way to perfect an existing test for non-A, non-

B hepatitis, based on the new knowledge of hepatitis C, to be used to screen the blood supply as is now done for the other forms of hepatitis. A vaccine, such as the one that already exists for hepatitis B, could be developed in a number of years, according to researchers.

Delta hepatitis can be prevented by vaccinating susceptible persons with hepatitis B vaccine. However, no simple method exists to protect hepatitis B carriers from delta superinfection.

Herpes

What is herpes?

There are at least seventy varieties of herpes viruses—most of which attack only animals. The herpes virus is large in relation to other viruses, highly complex in structure, and surrounded by what appears to be a protective envelope. The most common herpes viruses among humans are herpes simplex virus type I (HSV-1) and herpes simplex virus type II (HSV-2). Herpes simplex type I usually inhabits the head and is the cause of most cold sores, while type II usually occurs below the waist and is responsible for 80 percent of venereal herpes.

Three other types of herpes viruses afflict human beings: the varicella-zoster virus, which causes chicken pox and shingles; the Epstein-Barr virus, which causes mononucleosis; and cytomegalovirus (CMV), the most common source of fetal infections and the cause of hepatitis and pneumonialike illnesses in children and adults. Some researchers have speculated that herpes blisters in the stomach or intestines may precipitate ulcers.

Following are a few of the unsolved questions about herpes:

What happens to the virus when it lies latent in the body?
Why doesn't the immune system eradicate the virus?
Are portions of its DNA found in latently infected cells?
Has the virus somehow been incorporated into the host cells' chromosomes?
Does some irritant reactivate the virus?
Does the release of prostaglandins reactivate the virus?

Who can get herpes simplex?

Anyone is susceptible to herpes simplex—and no one ever really recovers from it. Anyone who contracts herpes virus is recurrently capable of spreading the virus. About a third of those who do contract herpes virus never get recurrences and are not considered infectious. For both genital and oral herpes virus, prevention is an important factor. Once a person has acquired a herpes virus, he or she should be extremely careful to avoid spreading the virus to uninfected parts of the body or transmitting the virus to uninfected persons. The virus is infectious when blisters or sores are present—until the sores are completely healed. It takes only one virus to cause infection—and the virus is so powerful that a person can become infected from a particle on an inanimate object. The virus has been proven to live for as long as 72 hours on a piece of cotton gauze, though the virus can be destroyed by boiling, alcohol, and lipid solvents of ether or chloroform. People with mild herpes lesions or with lesions hidden inside the body can pass the virus on to others without even knowing they have the disease.

> The ancient Greeks are responsible for naming herpes. The word *herpes*, from the Greek verb meaning *to creep*, describes herpes infection perfectly: sores that seem to creep over the surface of the skin. The early Romans knew about herpes, too. Nearly 2000 years ago, Roman Emperor Tiberius attempted to curb an epidemic of cold sores by outlawing kissing at public ceremonies and rituals. In 1886, two French physicians published the first comprehensive medical review of genital herpes.

How is herpes simplex transmitted?
Doctors suspect that the herpes simplex virus enters the body through the mucous membranes and soft tissues of the mouth or genitals, or through cuts or abrasions of the skin. Once established, the virus invades the cells of lower layers of the skin and begins to multiply. Some of the viruses enter the tiny endings of the sensory nerves and advance up the nerve to reside in the nerve-cell body. In facial herpes, the virus settles in the trigeminal ganglia, in nerve tissues near the cheekbone. Genital herpes find a home in the sacral ganglia in nerve tissue outside the spinal canal.

Facial herpes can be spread by kissing; genital herpes can be spread by sexual contact when the sores are present. When the sores aren't present, the disease does not spread. Sores that occur internally and cannot be seen make it difficult to determine when the disease is present. Autopsy studies show that at least 50 percent of Americans may harbor latent herpes viruses at the base of the brain and that 10 to 15 percent may harbor such viruses in the base of the spine.

What are the symptoms of herpes simplex I?

Herpes simplex I usually inhabits the head and is the cause of most cold sores. This type, which is usually not connected with sexual contact, can also infect the genitals, but when the virus causes genital sores, they are not likely to recur. Herpes simplex I is readily transmitted from one body part to another. The eyes, for example, can be infected simply by rubbing them after touching an infected area.

What are the symptoms of herpes simplex II?

Herpes simplex II is the type of herpes virus that causes the much-discussed and troublesome near-epidemic venereal disease called genital herpes. This form of the disease usually occurs below the waist and is most often spread through sexual intercourse. It is seen with increasing frequency in the 20–29 age group. It is more likely to cause recurrent infections than herpes simplex I.

What is the difference between primary and nonprimary genital herpes?

Primary first-episode herpes is the condition in which no herpes antibody is found, meaning that the person has never been exposed to the virus before. Usually, the course of this type of herpes tends to be more severe and of longer duration, since the body has no defense against the virus. The disease is referred to as nonprimary first-episode genital herpes when the herpes antibody is found. This antibody can be to type I or type II or both—and can result from infection with type I in fever blisters or from asymptomatic infection with type II in the genital area. Cases of primary genital herpes are more likely to develop complications such as aseptic meningitis, urinary retention, or whitlow—the inflammation of the end of a finger or toe.

What happens when herpes recurs?

Recurrent disease occurs because of the persistence of the herpes simplex virus in the ganglion (nerve cells) and is the result of reactivation of this virus. Usually, the recurrence is a milder, shorter illness than the first episode, and patients say they can feel the symptoms from a few hours to a few days before blistering occurs from itching and tingling sensations in the genital area. The duration of the viral shedding and healing time is much shorter than in the first episode. The average duration of first-episode disease is 21 days, compared with 10 days for recurrent disease.

How is herpes simplex virus treated?
Although there is currently no vaccine to prevent the acquisition of the virus, a new drug, acyclovir (Zovirax), is an effective treatment. In first-episode herpes, topical acyclovir shortens viral shedding, promotes healing, hastens crusting, and shortens the duration of the disease. Intravenous dosages of acyclovir are sometimes given to treat severe primary herpes. The following suggestions have also been helpful in managing herpes:

Use a hair dryer on the cool setting to help dry lesions and promote healing.
Take aspirin for pain.
Gently wash lesions with mild soap and running water and pat dry to keep clean and to aid drying.
Take sitz baths to help ease discomfort if pain is severe.
Avoid wearing tight pants or undergarments made of nylon.

How does acyclovir work?
Acyclovir is a chemical that imitates one of the building blocks of herpes' DNA. It mimics the virus so effectively that the virus tries to use the drug to reproduce itself. Since that does not work, the virus ultimately destroys itself. The drug can be taken orally and, according to doctors who prescribe it, up to five capsules a day can avoid all recurrences. The doctors note, however, that the drug is not a cure and that flare-ups will return if the medication is stopped. The long-term side effects of acyclovir are still unclear.

If a pregnant woman has genital herpes, can her unborn baby contract it?
The greatest risk for the baby is when the mother becomes in-

fected for the first time during a pregnancy, because the virus may get into the bloodstream and be passed to the infant. That does not happen very often.

Most pregnant women who have herpes deliver normal babies. Doctors guard against exposing the baby to active herpes infection during passage through the birth canal by examining specimens, sampling birth canal cells, and testing blood for antibodies beginning with the eighth month of pregnancy. If the studies are negative when it's time to deliver the baby, a vaginal delivery can be attempted. If the tests show active infection, a cesarean section is performed.

What is the relationship between genital herpes and cervical cancer?

There is an association between the two, according to research, but no cause-and-effect relationship has been proven. Not all women with genital herpes develop cervical cancer; however, more women who have genital herpes develop cervical cancer than those who do not have herpes. Studies have shown that women with genital herpes were almost four times more likely to have cervical cancer than the average woman. Though statistical and clinical relationships between herpes and cervical cancer have been documented, science is at a loss to demonstrate that the virus is responsible for the cancer. The link between papilloma virus and cancer of the cervix is now stronger than that between herpes and cervical cancer.

What is herpes encephalitis?

Herpes encephalitis is a complication of herpes that occurs if the brain becomes infected. An extremely rare disorder, it occurs when a virus present at sites on the face, lips, or mouth travels to the temporal lobe of the brain along nerve pathways from the trigeminal ganglion. Antiviral drugs can help prevent damage if the condition is treated in time.

What is herpes keratitis?

When the herpes virus affects the eye, the condition is known as herpes keratitis. The eyes are seldom the site of initial infection, but in rare cases the virus can travel directly from the trigeminal ganglion to the eye. The virus infection can cause lesions on the eye, which may result in partial or complete vision impairment. If treated in time, antiviral drugs can help prevent damage.

What is the role of idoxuridine in treating viral eye infections?

Idoxuridine is an antiviral ointment used in the treatment of viral eye infections—especially herpes keratitis. Idoxuridine irreversibly inhibits the virus replication by penetrating the host cell and inhibiting DNA synthesis.

Chicken Pox and Shingles

What causes chicken pox?

Chicken pox (also known as varicella) is a common infectious disease of children. It is caused by a virus closely related to the one that causes herpes and herpes zoster (shingles). It is one of the most highly contagious diseases of childhood, characterized by raised pimplelike bumps on the skin which develop translucent blisters that crust over and eventually disappear. One attack usually confers lifelong immunity.

What causes shingles?

Shingles and chicken pox are caused by the same virus, herpes zoster. People with herpes zoster transmit virus to produce chicken pox in the nonimmune. Shingles arise only in those who carry a dormant varicella zoster virus (chicken pox) and cannot be caught from another person. While young people do develop shingles, the disease most often strikes in later years, usually after age 50. However, children and adults whose immune systems are weakened, or who are taking anticancer drugs that suppress the immune system, are more likely to develop shingles.

Is shingles contagious?

Unlike chicken pox, which is a highly contagious disease, shingles is not transmitted by contact with an infected individual. In order to develop shingles, a person must already have had a case of chicken pox and harbor the virus in his or her nervous system. When activated, the virus travels down nerves to the skin, causing the painful shingles rash. Because the shingles rash contains active virus particles, however, a person who has never had chicken pox can contract chicken pox by exposure to the shingles rash.

Are there any drugs available to help treat shingles?

One drug in limited use is vidarabine. This drug interferes with the ability of the herpes zoster virus to make new genetic material and thus prevents the virus from reproducing and spreading in the body. Early treatment with vidarabine decreased the duration of shingles in a group of eighty-seven patients with deficient immune responses. Acyclovir is also being tested on zoster patients. Once activated by a chemical produced by the virus, acyclovir is able to destroy a vital chemical that the virus needs in order to reproduce. Interferon is also being tested and has been found to lessen pain and reduce complications.

Is there a relationship between shingles (herpes zoster) and cancer?

A number of studies attempted to determine if the risk of developing cancer increases among people who have had shingles. Although the studies were not conclusive, the largest study—in Rochester, Minnesota—indicates that the incidence of cancer during the first year and the first 5 years after an attack of herpes zoster is the same as the incidence in the general population.

Why aren't children vaccinated against chicken pox?

Some scientists have been reluctant to consider a chicken pox vaccine because they fear the long-range future consequences of such a vaccine. Chicken pox virus lurks in the body after the illness passes, sometimes reawakening in later life to cause shingles. It is unknown whether the vaccine virus would produce shingles, as chicken pox does, or whether it would have other, as yet unknown side effects. Since normally there are few serious complications from chicken pox, and since the chicken pox virus is unusually complex, many doctors feel that it is unwise to vaccinate against an illness as mild as chicken pox.

What is the danger of chicken pox in children with cancer?

Among normal children, chicken pox accounts for fewer than fifty deaths a year in the United States. However, for children who have leukemia or related forms of cancer and are being treated with anticancer drugs that suppress the patient's normal defenses, chicken pox can be a life-threatening disease. Shingles may follow chicken pox, within months or a year, in immunosuppressed children; therefore, precautions are important.

What chicken pox vaccines are used for children with cancer?
There are two vaccines against chicken pox, primarily used for
children with leukemia who have been exposed to chicken pox.
ZIG (zoster immune globulin), a concentrate, is administered intra-
muscularly rather than intravenously. ZIP (zoster immune plasma)
is obtained from patients who are recovering from a herpes zoster
(shingles) infection. They are equally effective for the prevention of
chicken pox in immunosuppressed children, and should be administered within 72 hours of exposure to the chicken pox. There is a
greater risk of hepatitis complications with ZIP than with ZIG.
Interferon and several new vaccines are being tested.

Epstein-Barr Virus

What is the Epstein-Barr virus?
The Epstein-Barr virus is a herpeslike virus. Most Americans are
harmlessly infected with the virus during childhood and are immune from further infections. Epstein-Barr virus can cause infectious mononucleosis in young adults who escaped childhood
infection. It has also been associated with Burkitt's lymphoma,
normally a childhood cancer in Africa. Almost everyone who
develops Burkitt's lymphoma also has been infected by the virus, but only one child in 2000 who has been infected by the virus
develops the cancer, suggesting that other unknown factors are
also involved.

What is chronic Epstein-Barr virus syndrome?
First described in the medical literature in 1948, chronic Epstein-
Barr virus syndrome describes patients who have had infectious
mononucleosis and whose symptoms have persisted for a year or
longer. In many cases, the syndrome first appears after an attack
of infectious mononucleosis, which produces nearly identical
symptoms. The virus persists for years in an activated form, causing continuous or recurring symptoms of chronic fatigue, aches
and pains, loss of appetite, and depression. Patients feel as though
they are having a chronic or relapsing case of the flu, with muscle
aches, sore throat, swollen glands, low-grade fevers, and extraor-
dinary fatigue. In some, the symptoms are present most of the
time. In others, they come and go, recurring severely one to six
times a year with fatigue persisting between attacks. Some patients are diagnosed as neurotic, with later evidence that they are

suffering from the effects of the virus, which can produce symptoms of depression and anxiety.

There is presently no diagnostic test for chronic Epstein-Barr virus syndrome. Nor is there any remedy for the condition, although several are under investigation. Many doctors find that simply knowing there is a medical explanation for the symptoms—that it is not a neurotic reaction—helps many patients. Scientists warn that children with this disorder may be misdiagnosed and treated with antibiotics or injections of immunoglobulin, both of which can produce adverse effects.

What is mononucleosis?

Mononucleosis is a viral infectious disease that usually occurs in people between the ages of 15 and 25. It is often called "the kissing disease," supposedly because it is believed to be transmitted through close contact. Symptoms range from barely noticeable to severe and debilitating—with fever, weakness, sore throat, and swollen glands being common. Mononucleosis is caused by the Epstein-Barr (EB) herpes virus, which causes a large identifiable mononuclear (single-nucleus) white blood cell to appear in the blood. Presently there is no vaccine available for mononucleosis.

CMV

What is cytomegalovirus?

Cytomegalovirus, known as CMV, attacks 1 to 2 percent of newborns and causes mental retardation in about 2500 infants per year. CMV live-virus vaccines against this rare disease are being tested in the laboratory. The virus occasionally causes hepatitis or Paul Bunnell negative infectious mononucleosis, but it is most commonly confined to pregnant women. It is a virus that can cross the placenta. Maternal antibodies do not protect the fetus from infection, although they do lessen the risk of damage to newborns.

Are there differences in the incidence of congenital CMV infection in different socioeconomic groups?

Yes. There are considerable differences due to geographic and racial as well as socioeconomic conditions.

Measles: Rubeola, Rubella, Roseola

What causes measles?

Measles (rubeola) is caused by a viral infection. It isn't really the virus that creates the symptoms that characterize measles. Rather, it is the natural immunological counterattack that causes the symptoms we see. The virus multiplies in the body for a number of days, during which the patient exhibits no effects. Then the fever, red skin rash, cough, itching, redness of the eyes, and swelling of the face occur. The disease we call measles is actually the immune process bringing the infection under control. Once the virus has attacked the body, the body becomes immune forever.

Does measles sometimes impair or kill?

For reasons that are still obscure, serious complications develop in one out of every 1000 cases of measles. A dangerous inflammation of brain tissue is sometimes the aftermath of the measles infection. Other more deadly aftereffects include a rare disease referred to by a variety of names but most often known as SSPE (*subacute sclerosing panencephalitis*). The symptoms include a deterioriation of the child's intellect as well as strange periodic muscle spasms of the arms, legs, and trunk. The loss of mental and physical skills becomes progressively more pronounced, and the child usually dies within months. This disease was once thought to be caused by a rare hereditary defect. It is now known to be a result of the measles virus.

Is there a measles vaccine?

A live-virus measles vaccine is available and immunizes practically 100 percent of susceptible individuals. Consequently, this highly contagious, once-prevalent childhood disease—which used to appear in epidemics, often in wintertime—is now rarely seen. Passive immunization can be conferred by doses of gamma globulin. Many doctors reserve the use of gamma globulin for those patients for whom live measles-virus vaccine may involve some risk, such as children with leukemia, Hodgkin's disease, or malignant tumors.

What is rubella?

Rubella, more commonly known as German or 3-day measles, is a viral disease that has an incubation period of 2 to 3 weeks. A usually harmless disease, which is recognizable by a flat pink rash that covers the body, rubella can be catastrophic for the pregnant mother and the fetus. Though the pregnant mother may not be very sick, the developing baby can become mentally retarded or deaf or suffer heart damage as a result of the mother's rubella infection. Rubella results in abnormalities in 50 percent of fetuses whose mothers are infected during the first month of pregnancy, and in 15 percent of fetuses whose mothers are infected during the third month. Every woman of childbearing age should be tested to see if she is immune to rubella. If she is not, there is a vaccine available that should be given when the patient is not pregnant or likely to become pregnant for 3 months.

Is roseola different from measles (rubeola)?

Yes. Roseola, a disease that is probably caused by a virus, produces a rash and is sometimes confused with measles (rubeola). It is most often seen in children between the ages of 1 and 3. Fever, usually over 103 degrees, is the initial symptom, though the child usually feels well except for a depressed appetite. After 3 days, the temperature usually drops to normal, at which time the child sometimes becomes much more irritable. After 24 hours without fever, a generalized fine, flat pink rash of the trunk is noted. The rash lasts for about 2 days. The cause of roseola has not been conclusively determined, and there is no vaccine against it.

Mumps

Is mumps caused by a viral infection?

Yes. The virus can invade many tissues in the body and can cause swelling, fever, headache, stomachache, and vomiting. The most common symptom is the swelling of the parotid saliva glands, in the hollow just under the earlobe or in the lower part of the jawbone. The swelling may begin on one side first, sometimes spreading to the opposite side. Mumps may spread to the testicles of men or boys who have reached puberty. Complications of mumps include meningitis and encephalitis. It may spread to the pancreas or to the ovaries.

A live-virus vaccine is available for mumps. A skin test is also available to determine if a person is immune or susceptible—especially important if an adult male is exposed to mumps, since the disease can be painful. A mumps immune globulin is available to help lessen the symptoms in adults.

Papilloma (warts, condyloma)

What causes warts?
Warts are caused by a papilloma virus that takes over skin cells and makes them grow to suit the virus. Each infected cell bulges with virus particles. Antibodies develop to the wart virus, and in most children warts spontaneously drop off within a few months to a few years. Some people, perhaps because of low immunity to this particular virus, have more trouble with warts than others.

What is papilloma virus?
The papilloma virus has been recognized since the 1930s but has been very difficult to study because it cannot be grown in laboratory tissue cultures. Recently, the development of molecular biology has provided the means for identifying the virus in human and animal tissues by detecting chemical traces of the virus in the cells it infects.

Originally the human papilloma virus was thought of as a single entity; however, the new chemical research has demonstrated that there are many different types associated with different effects on the human body. A few years ago, nine of them had been identified. Today more than thirty different human papilloma viruses have been categorized.

What are the different kinds of human papilloma viruses?
Type 1 causes plantar warts that grow on the soles of the feet. The warts are essentially harmless but are painful.

Type 2 causes common warts that usually appear on the hands.

Type 3 causes flat warts of the face, found particularly in young people.

Type 4 causes plantar warts on the hands and plantar warts on the feet.

Type 6 causes condyloma, a kind of wart of the female genital tract.

Type 7 causes warts in butchers and other meat handlers. These warts can grow rapidly and incapacitate the patients.

Type 11 causes an uncommon disease involving fast-growing warts on the larynx, especially in young children. The warts need to be removed every 2 months or even more frequently, since they can block the flow of air to the lungs. Sometimes the growths simply shrink in time.

Type 13 causes flat wartlike lesions of the mouth.

Types 6, 11, 16, and 18 are found in genital warts.

Types 16 and 18 have been linked to cervical cancers.

Types 5, 8, 9, 10, 12, 14, 15, 17, 19, and 26 have been associated with a rare skin disease called epidermodysplasia verruciformis, which has also been linked with the later development of cancer.

Do the papilloma viruses cause cancer?

Although most of the papilloma viruses in humans cause noncancerous growths, several scientists feel that the evidence is strong that some of the papilloma viruses are linked to cancers of the cervix and vulva and with a rare kind of skin cancer. They feel the findings for the papilloma virus are far stronger than those linking genital cancers to herpes.

In women studied at Georgetown University, traces of the same papilloma virus could be found in the original cancers and in distant metastatic growths that arose from those cancers. The evidence showed presence of the same virus in precancerous, cancerous, and metastatic tissues.

Scientists at the University of Minnesota studying a rare, genetically based, wartlike skin disease (epidermodysplasia verruciformis) found some 30 percent of patients developed skin cancer, apparently as a progression of the skin disease. Traces of papilloma viruses were found in all the cancers of this type studied by the researchers.

Efforts are under way to develop a vaccine against the virus, but it will likely be several years before that is accomplished.

Do animals also get papilloma viruses?

Yes. Humans aren't the only species susceptible to warts. Papilloma viruses pervade the animal kingdom. Deer, sheep, dogs, birds, and rabbits are susceptible to warts. Warts the size of bowling balls have been treated in cows. Horses can get papilloma infections of the muzzle. And, as in humans, the virus is known to cause cancers in animals.

What is condyloma virus?

A major cause of concern in today's sexually active population is the condyloma virus, a type of papilloma virus. Researchers have found evidence of cluster cases of a condyloma-related, precancerous cervical condition in women. Genital warts are caused by the sexually transmitted condyloma virus. If not detected and dealt with early, the condition can progress to cervical cancer. High-risk groups include women who were younger than 20 when they first had intercourse, women who have had multiple (more than three) partners, and women who have had intercourse with a man who has had multiple sex partners. Risks increase fourfold for smokers. The symptoms of the condyloma virus are the appearance of flat, projecting, or inverted warts in the genital area, usually within 3 months of exposure. The warts often appear in clusters, have the texture of cauliflower, and are painless. Presence of the virus can be difficult to detect in men, because many of the warts are very small and there is no comparable test to the Pap smear for men. Like herpes simplex virus II, the condyloma virus appears to be a cancer promoter. The virus can be transmitted to a baby in the birth canal, and often it appears in the newborn in the form of laryngeal warts, which can cause breathing difficulties. Doctors feel that the use of condoms probably guards against most intravaginal, sexually transmitted diseases.

What is the treatment for condyloma viruses?
Sometimes they disappear without treatment. For those that don't, the disease is treated by a number of methods. The most common are topical chemical application, freezing with liquid nitrogen, burning out with lasers, or removing surgically. None of these treatments is always effective, and more than half the time the warts return. Interferon is being tested as a treatment for condylomas. In the trials, interferon has been given successfully to patients whose genital warts failed to respond to ordinary treatment.

AIDS

What are the HTLV viruses?
HTLV stands for *h*uman *T*-cell *l*eukemia-lymphoma *v*iruses, a family of retroviruses that have been identified in human tissues. Three have been found. HTLV-I is strongly associated with a form of adult T-cell leukemia-lymphoma that is unusual in the United States but fairly common in other parts of the world, such as southwest Japan, the Caribbean basin, parts of Africa, and South and Central

America. HTLV-II is weakly linked with hairy-cell leukemia. HTLV-III is strongly implicated in the development of *a*cquired *i*mmune *d*eficiency *s*yndrome (AIDS).

The three types of HTLV share these features:

- They are acquired from outside the cells by infection.
- They bud from cell membranes. The virus completes its life cycle inside the cell it infects, producing progeny viruses that can leave the infected cell.
- They have an affinity for lymphocytes, particularly immune system T4 helper cells that boost the body defenses against infections.
- They have a major core protein, known as p24, that is different from the core proteins of other animal retroviruses.
- They all have similar major regions of gene chromosomes, confirming that the three viruses belong to the same family. One, however, performs differently, which may explain why two are associated with T-cell cancers and the third is linked with an immune suppressive disease.
- They all appear to be of African origin.

What is AIDS?

AIDS (*a*cquired *i*mmune *d*eficiency *s*yndrome) is a serious condition characterized by a defect in natural immunity against disease and the presence of the HTLV-III virus. People who suffer from AIDS become susceptible to a variety of rare illnesses. The two diseases most commonly found in AIDS patients are pneumocystis carinii pneumonia, a lung infection caused by a parasite, and Kaposi's sarcoma, a rare form of cancer or tumor of the blood-vessel walls. These two diseases are not usually found in people whose immune systems are normal, and if they should occur in those with normal immune systems, they are usually mild. Physicians have recently reported links between the AIDS virus in homosexual men and another kind of cancer, a severe form of malignant lymphoma. Of twenty lymphoma patients tested by medical scientists at the University of Southern California, fifteen had antibodies to HTLV-III, indicating they had been or were infected with the virus.

What are the symptoms of AIDS?

Symptoms may include fever; night sweats; enlarged lymph nodes in the neck, armpits, or groin; unexplained weight loss; yeast infections; diarrhea; persistent coughs; fatigue; and loss of appetite.

Who gets AIDS?

Nearly 95 percent of AIDS cases have occurred in people belonging to one of six distinct groups. Sexually active homosexual and bisexual men with multiple sex partners account for more than 70 percent of all reported cases. Seventeen percent of the reported cases involve present or past abusers of intravenous drugs. Nearly 2 percent of AIDS cases are related to blood transfusions; another 1 percent of victims are steady sexual partners (male and female) of persons with AIDS or persons in groups at high risk for AIDS. Hemophiliacs make up 0.7 percent of AIDS victims. Infants and children who have developed AIDS or a syndrome similar to AIDS may have been exposed to AIDS before or during birth or have a history of transfusions.

How is AIDS diagnosed?

The diagnosis of AIDS depends on the presence of opportunistic diseases—serious illnesses that would not be a threat to anyone whose immune system was functioning normally. Certain tests that demonstrate damage to various parts of the immune system, such as specific types of white blood cells, support the diagnosis. The presence of opportunistic diseases plus a positive test for antibodies to HTLV-III can also make possible a diagnosis of AIDS.

As with most other infections, there is no single test for diagnosing AIDS. There is now a test for antibodies to the virus that causes AIDS. Presence of HTLV-III antibodies means that a person has been infected with the AIDS virus. It does not tell whether the person is still infected. The antibody test is used to screen donated blood and plasma and to assist in preventing cases of AIDS resulting from blood transfusions or use of blood products, such as factor VIII needed by men with hemophilia. The test is also available through private physicians, most state or local health departments, and other sites.

How is AIDS transmitted?

AIDS is transmitted primarily through sexual contact, through needle sharing, or through blood from a person who has AIDS. To date, most of the cases have involved homosexual and bisexual men with multiple sex partners. AIDS has also been traced to intravenous drug abusers, leading investigators to suspect that AIDS is transmitted by blood on contaminated needles that have been shared.

Other evidence of transmission of AIDS through blood products was found in hemophilia patients receiving large amounts of factor VIII, a clotting substance. AIDS may also be transmitted from infected mother to infant before, during, or shortly after birth.

How contagious is AIDS?

No cases have been found where AIDS has been transmitted by casual or normal household contact with AIDS patients or persons in the high-risk groups. A large study conducted by Dr. Gerald H. Friedland of Montefiore Hospital, Bronx, New York, reported in the *New England Journal of Medicine*, indicates that the risk of transmitting AIDS through normal household contact is "virtually nonexistent." Although HTLV-III virus has been found, through rarely, in saliva of some persons at risk for AIDS, there have been no cases in which saliva was shown to be the route of transmission. In one case, the virus was found in the tears of an AIDS patient. Ambulance drivers, police, and firefighters who have assisted AIDS patients, and nurses, doctors, and health care personnel have not developed AIDS from exposure to AIDS patients. There have been no known cases of transmission through food or water or through the air by coughing or sneezing. Although casual contact with AIDS patients' tears has not been associated with the syndrome, the National Institutes of Health has recommended that direct contact with the tears of AIDS patients, including contact during routine ophthalmologic procedures, should be minimized. Safety procedures should be followed carefully when handling any blood and tissue samples from patients with AIDS.

How long after exposure to HTLV-III does a person develop AIDS?

The time between infection with HTLV-III virus and the onset of symptoms seems to range from about 6 months to 5 years and possibly longer. Not everyone exposed to the virus develops AIDS.

Can the AIDS virus live for a long time outside the body?

The virus cannot reproduce outside a living cell but may survive for a period of days outside the body—in bodily fluid—under the right temperature and light conditions.

How do children and babies get AIDS?

They get AIDS in four ways: from blood transfusions, by the virus crossing into the fetus's blood through the placenta, through exposure to an infected mother's blood during childbirth, or through the breast milk of an infected mother.

How is AIDS treated?

Currently there are no antiviral drugs available anywhere that have been proven to cure AIDS, although the search for such a drug is being pursued vigorously. Some drugs inhibit the AIDS virus, but these do not lead to clinical improvement.

Although no treatment has yet been successful in restoring the immune system of an AIDS patient to normal function, doctors have had some success in using drugs, radiation, and surgery to treat the various illnesses suffered by AIDS patients. Therapeutic agents are needed for all stages of AIDS infections, to block action of the virus once infection has occurred and to build up immunity in patients who have developed AIDS symptoms. Eventually, a combination chemotherapy to combat the virus and restore the immune system may be the most effective therapy. Pneumocystis carinii, for example, can be treated with antibiotics. Interferon, a virus-fighting protein produced naturally by the body, has been used with some success against Kaposi's sarcoma. Natural and recombinant interleukin preparations are being used in an attempt to repair the immunologic deficiencies in AIDS patients.

Is the disease worse in pregnant women?

It seems to be. According to researchers at the Downstate Medical Center in Brooklyn who followed the syndrome in three pregnant women who presumably got AIDS from intravenous drug use, the disease took its fatal course unusually quickly. All three died during their initial hospital admission for AIDS. Two of the three delivered their babies, who are alive and AIDS free, before dying. The physicians do not know whether the disease was diagnosed late because the early AIDS symptoms were passed off as side effects of pregnancy or whether the slightly lowered immunity of pregnant women could have offered less resistance to it.

Can AIDS cause brain damage?

Yes. Researchers have found that the AIDS virus infects cells within the human brain and central nervous system, resulting in loss of intellect and memory, confusion, seizures, and other mental illnesses. Some brains of AIDS patients are shrunken, with their interior spaces dilated. Scientists believe that the blood-brain barrier, a feature of the circulatory system that prevents many substances, including drugs, from getting into the brain, could be providing a sanctuary for the AIDS viruses. They feel that even if treatments could be devised to stop a virus infection and to allow the immune system to rebuild itself, brain damage is likely to be permanent.

Can the hepatitis vaccine spread AIDS?

Because it is made from the plasma of carriers of hepatitis B, many of whom may also be in the population at high risk for AIDS, the question has arisen. However, the procedures used in the manufacture of hepatitis B vaccine inactivate viruses from every known group. Therefore, the risk of vaccine-induced infection by any transmissible agent that might cause AIDS is extremely remote. In addition, the blood tests being administered to detect antibodies to the AIDS virus in the blood of hepatitis B carriers will further ensure the safety of the vaccine.

What is the blood test for AIDS?

The blood test, though it cannot detect the AIDS virus, can reveal whether a person's immune system has begun producing blood antibodies to attack the virus in the bloodstream. The presence of antibodies only means that the person tested has been exposed to the virus. It does not mean that the person will develop AIDS or that he or she is infectious. The test may also lead to earlier diagnosis of the disease.

Are there different strains of AIDS virus?

The AIDS virus is known variously as HTLV-III (*human T-lymphotropic virus, type III*), LAV (*lymphadenopathy-associated virus*), or ARV (*AIDS-related virus*), depending upon which scientific team has discovered it. Most experts agree that it is all the same virus, although there has been variability in the different viral specimens found in patients. It seems to be changing significantly as it infects the U.S. population, a moving target, complicating efforts to combat the virus with a vaccine. Researchers feel that the virus may be escaping detection by the immune system by changing its genetic identity.

When were the first cases of AIDS diagnosed in the United States?

In mid-1981, five cases of pneumocystis carinii pneumonia, an unusual disease caused by a parasitic organism, were reported by the Centers for Disease Control in Atlanta. All five were found in previously healthy, sexually active, young homosexual men from Los Angeles, with no history of immune suppression. This type of pneumonia is almost always seen in immune-suppressed individuals. Further testing revealed that three of the men had abnormally depressed immune systems.

At about the same time, 26 cases of Kaposi's sarcoma, a rare skin cancer seen in elderly men of Jewish or Mediterranean descent or in recipients of kidney transplants, were reported. Again, the men were young and homosexual, this time from New York as well as Los Angeles. By late August, less then 3 months after the first report, the Centers for Disease Control knew of more than 100 cases where helper T cells had been nearly wiped out. With time, other types of unusual viral, fungal, or parasitic infections were being diagnosed in young homosexuals with similar immune defects. The first report on AIDS was published in the *New England Journal of Medicine* in December of 1981.

Is AIDS found in every state in the United States?
Yes. Every state has reported at least one case, although 36 percent of the cases come from New York and about 23 percent from California. AIDS cases have also been reported from more than thirty-five other countries.

Can AIDS be prevented?
Yes. Cases of AIDS related to medical use of blood or blood products are being prevented by use of HTLV-III antibody screening tests before blood is accepted for transfusion. Members of high-risk groups are being tested and asked voluntarily not to donate blood. Heat treatment of factor VIII and other blood products is being used to help prevent AIDS in patients with hemophilia and other clotting disorders. There is no vaccine for AIDS itself. However, there is good reason to believe that individuals can reduce their risk of contracting AIDS by following existing recommendations, such as not having sexual contact with persons known or suspected of having AIDS or with multiple partners or with persons who have had multiple partners. Other recommendations include not abusing intravenous drugs, not sharing needles or syringes if using intravenous drugs, and not having sex with people who abuse intravenous drugs.

Polio

What is polio?
Poliomyelitis, also known as infantile paralysis, is a paralyzing disease of the nervous system. It is caused by a virus infection of the spinal cord and the motor cranial nerves. This dreaded

disease has been virtually eliminated by the use first of killed vaccine (Salk type), which was injected into patients, and more recently by the oral vaccines (Sabin type) containing living viruses. Once responsible for 35,000 cases of disease in the United States each year, polio epidemics were common each year until 1955, when the first vaccine was introduced. Prepared by Jonas E. Salk, the vaccine contained killed viruses of each of the three strains known to produce the disease.

What are the symptoms of polio?
The disease begins, like so many other infections, with a general sick feeling (malaise), fever, and headache. There may be vomiting, constipation, or a little diarrhea. In about 80 percent of cases, polio victims survive without paralysis. In severe attacks, however, there is pain and stiffness in the neck and paralysis develops. Limbs as well as respiratory muscles can be affected—with permanent, disabling results. In severe cases, cranial nerves and the spinal cord are also involved.

Multiple Sclerosis

What is multiple sclerosis?
Multiple sclerosis (MS) is a crippling disease of the nervous system. Although its cause has not been definitively established, the disease is believed to result from a slow-virus infection. It affects people between the ages of 20 and 50, and its onset can easily be mistaken for other conditions. The patient commonly complains initially of tingling in a limb or clumsiness, which seems to disappear. Symptoms vary depending on the site of the plaques (areas where nerve fibers have been damaged), but blurring of vision, clumsiness of movement, tingling, and patches of numbness in various parts of the body usually recur. In the early stages of the disease, symptoms may disappear, only to reappear again. The condition usually worsens and becomes chronic. Multiple sclerosis affects about 250,000 Americans. About 8800 are afflicted every year, most of them young or middle-aged adults.

What produces the crippling effects of multiple sclerosis?
In somewhat the same way that an electrical wire is protected by insulation, the nerve fibers in the body are normally coated with a fatty protein material called myelin. In multiple sclerosis, the myelin surrounding the nerve fibers is randomly destroyed. This destruction interferes with the transmission of nerve signals to the

brain and spinal cord from the part of the body that has been attacked. The loss of the myelin from the white matter in the brain and spinal cord occurs in a sharply defined area, called a plaque, which looks like an inkblot and results in a firmer, rubbery texture to the tissue. For the most part these multiple sclerosis plaques still contain intact nerve fibers, but the fibers are stripped of myelin. Interestingly enough, function has sometimes returned even though obvious plaques are still present.

What causes multiple sclerosis?

The cause is unknown, but there are several theories. A slow-virus infection has been suspected. T-cell imbalance seems to play a key role in the disease, and certain T cells appear to be involved in the destruction of myelin. Patients with severe multiple sclerosis have subnormal T-cell levels and depleted suppressor cells. Healthy people and patients with other neurological disorders show no such variations in peripheral suppressor cells.

Preliminary findings, recently published in the British scientific journal *Nature*, suggest that multiple sclerosis is an infectious disease caused or, perhaps, triggered by an unidentified virus that appears related to one that causes a rare form of leukemia. Although the evidence does not prove a viral cause, it points to a virus whose traces have appeared only in patients with multiple sclerosis and which has not been linked to any other disease. The researchers—from the Wistar Institute in Philadelphia; the National Cancer Institute in Bethesda, Maryland; the University of Lund in Sweden; and the University of Miami—compared patients with multiple sclerosis and healthy people, looking for two signs of virus infection: a certain kind of antibody and traces of the genetic code carried by an invading virus that can splice its genes into those of a victim's cells. Sixty percent of the patients with multiple sclerosis had the antibodies, while none of the healthy people had them. The research suggests that the patients at some time had been infected with a particular virus. What the virus is, no one knows. The antibodies, however, were of the type detected by a test developed to find antibodies made to attack a leukemia virus known as HTLV-I.

What triggers flare-ups of multiple sclerosis?

Two studies recently published in the British journal *Lancet*, one by Dr. Steven Narod of the University of Ottawa and another by Dr. William A. Sibley of the University of Arizona, note that multiple sclerosis patients seem to have fewer viral diseases than healthy people but that when coldlike symptoms do occur, they often trigger new attacks of the multiple sclerosis. The Canadian study on nineteen patients found that 32 percent of their new attacks of the disease coincided with colds. The Arizona research, conducted over 8 years on 170 patients with multiple sclerosis and a comparison group of 134 healthy people, found that 27 percent of the MS flare-ups followed viral infections. Most of these minor illnesses included respiratory symptoms. The Arizona research also showed that patients with multiple sclerosis had 20 to 50 percent fewer common infections than healthy people. Those with the greatest disability had the fewest infections. One theory is that white blood cells that are intended to attack cold viruses become confused and attack nerve tissue as well. The damage appears to be the result of internal mistaken identity.

What research is being done on multiple sclerosis?

Researchers at Stanford University have been able to selectively suppress certain cells of the immune systems of mice to reverse the effects of an animal disease similar to multiple sclerosis. Dr. Lawrence Steinman and his colleagues stimulated the MS-like disease in mice and treated it with monoclonal antibodies directed against the white "helper T cells," which seem to be responsible for destroying the myelin sheaths that insulate nerve fibers. They reported that the antibodies injected into the mice prevented development of disease symptoms if given early, and reversed paralysis and other nerve impairment in more advanced cases.

Dr. Howard L. Weiner and his colleagues at Brigham and Women's Hospitals in Boston have been injecting patients with doses of monoclonal antibodies that zero in on T cells and destroy them. In about half of their patients on the investigational treatment, the disease seemed to be arrested and in some cases reversed for 6 months. The testing so far has been to see whether the therapy is safe and affects the disease. More elaborate studies using comparison groups over 3 to 5 years will be necessary before doctors know how well it works.

Is there any relationship between climate and multiple sclerosis?

Multiple sclerosis is more likely to occur in colder climates—and is clustered in specific areas. For instance, the incidence of the disease in Canada is more than twice that of the United States.

Among the spots where there is more concentration of multiple sclerosis are two in the eastern United States, two in Northern Ireland, two in England, one in Washington state, one in Finland, and one in Saskatchewan. Some researchers who are studying this disease are looking at environmental influences, such as the presence of toxins or normal chemicals encountered in daily life.

Other confounding facts about this disease are that people tend to suffer fewer symptoms in cold weather and that people with multiple sclerosis who are able to walk often lose that ability when they have a fever—indicating a temperature relationship. Dr. Floyd Davis and colleagues at Rush Medical College in Chicago have been working with a drug that mimics the effects of the cold on nerves. Early results show that the drug, 4-aminopridine, can improve symptoms of patients with particularly heat-sensitive multiple sclerosis.

Kuru

What is kuru?

In the 1950s, it seemed as though a small group of New Guinea natives, known as Fores, might all be doomed to die of a disease known as kuru. The victims, usually women or children, first became aware of the disease because of an unsteadiness in gait, sometimes preceded by headaches and pains in the arms and legs. Loss of coordination and tremors of the head and limbs, often aggravated by cold, made up the next phase. In later stages, the victims suffered from slurred speech, inability to control the eyes and limbs, and mental deterioration.

What causes kuru?

Dr. D. Carleton Gajdusek and his colleagues studied the strange disease and collected records of more than 1400 cases as the outbreak reached epidemic proportions. At first it was thought that kuru had genetic origins. It was determined that the disease had probably first appeared about 40 or 50 years earlier, and had spread gradually throughout the population. Researchers were unable to find any characteristic antibodies or abnormalities in the blood or lymph systems, and the disease didn't seem to be transmissible from person to person. Animal experiments, however, proved that injection of the filtered material from the brains of victims into chimpanzees caused kuru symptoms months after the injections. Furthermore, material from the brain of one chimpanzee proved capable of passing the disease along to others *only when injected.*

Further investigation into the Fore people's customs uncovered the fact that, at elaborate funeral ceremonies, the women of the tribe removed the brain of the dead person and the mourners shared in eating it. However, the disease was not spread simply by eating the brain tissue of the infected victim, for not every participant came down with kuru. It was found that the women who removed the brains for the ceremonial feast used razor-sharp bamboo slivers and tested the sharpness of slivers by pricking their own forearms. Children helped prepare the feasts, and it is believed that the virus was passed to them through the usual cuts and scrapes of childhood. The Fore people changed their funeral procedures shortly after the researchers visited the village, and the disease began to decline.

Most puzzling is the fact that an agent as potent and destructive as kuru seems to leave no immunologic traces of its presence. Several immune system diseases—two in animals, two in man—seem to fall into the same category. Kuru and Creutzfeldt-Jakob disease have been found in relatively few humans—but they display many of the same characteristics. Scrapie, a sheep affliction, and transmissible mink encephalopathy, a disease of ranch-bred mink, also are fatal, progressive illnesses that involve destruction of tissues in the brain and central nervous system. All appear to be caused by slow viruses, but their long period of latency and their resistance to agents that destroy most viruses place them among the most unusual and mysterious of viral diseases.

Creutzfeldt-Jakob Disease

What is Creutzfeldt-Jakob disease?

Creutzfeldt-Jakob disease is a rare, usually fatal illness, causing confusion, loss of memory, and diminishing intellectual judgment. The symptoms are similar to those of kuru in humans and scrapie in sheep. It is named after two doctors who, independently, found cases of the same disease in different places. Relatively few cases have been diagnosed, but the disease has been seen in Europe, Canada, and the United States. It is believed to have been responsible for the death of choreographer George Balanchine. Though its symptoms are similar to those of Alzheimer's disease, Creutzfeldt-Jakob disease progresses faster, resulting in death within months rather than years.

What research is being done on Creutzfeldt-Jakob disease and scrapie?

Research, announced in the January 1985 issue of the *New England Journal of Medicine,* indicates that a recently identified class of infectious agents, smaller than viruses, called prions, are the cause of Creutzfeldt-Jakob disease. Researchers from the University of California's Berkeley and San Francisco campuses say they have conclusive evidence that prions are the cause of the condition. In 1982 it was discovered that prions cause scrapie, a degenerative neurological disease of sheep.

There is no evidence that Creutzfeldt-Jakob disease is transmissible from human to human except accidentally—perhaps through an inoculation into the brain as the result of a contaminated cornea transplant or contaminated electrodes implanted in the brain during a diagnostic test. Studies show that the brains of patients with Creutzfeldt-Jakob disease contain clusters of prions that have the same molecular structure and other characteristics as the scrapie prions. These clusters have not been found in normal brains nor in brains from victims of other kinds of senility, including Alzheimer's disease.

Is there a relationship between natural human growth hormone and Creutzfeldt-Jakob disease?

Yes, there is. Four children who had been treated for years with natural human growth hormone to prevent severe dwarfism died in a 10-month period in 1985 from Creutzfeldt-Jakob disease. The deaths were particularly alarming because Creutzfeldt-Jakob disease is extraordinarily rare, is always fatal, and is known to be transmissible by material from an infected brain. The time lapse between infection and disease can be many years. Experts say there is only about one case of Creutzfeldt-Jakob disease among a million people. The risk of its occurring in a person under 40 years old is only about one in 100 million. Three of the deaths were among the 11,000 young Americans who have received the hormone, and one was among those who had taken it in England, with all victims in their twenties and thirties. The odds against this happening by chance are astronomical.

Children who cannot make their own human growth hormone need injections of the substance two or three times every week through puberty in order to avoid dwarfism. The only source of human growth hormone has been the pituitary glands of people who have died. Allocation of the hormone, purified and distributed through the National Hormone and Pituitary Program financed by the federal government, was halted following the deaths. It is expected that the Food and Drug Administration will approve an artificially produced growth hormone in the near future.

Alzheimer's Disease

What causes Alzheimer's disease?

No one yet knows what causes Alzheimer's disease, named for the German neurologist Alois Alzheimer, who in 1906 found clumps of twisted nerve-cell fibers, called neurofibrillary tangles, in the brain of a 51-year-old woman. Several theories as to its origins are now being investigated. Some researchers believe that the disease may have not one, but several interlocking causes, such as genes, viruses, or toxins.

It is believed that inheritance plays a role in about 10 to 15 percent of Alzheimer's cases and that children of patients have a 50 percent risk of developing the disease. The younger the relative is when he gets the disease, the greater the risk for others in the family. Another indication of genetic involvement lies in the fact that virtually anyone with Down's syndrome (a form of mental retardation caused by an extra chromosome in the body's cells) develops what seems to be Alzheimer's after the age of 35 or 40.

Some researchers theorize a viral connection, based on experimental evidence that putting diseased brain extracts into healthy cultures can lead to the formation of neurofibrillary tangles. This brain-to-brain transmission of disease is a characteristic of other neurological disorders known to be caused by a virus, such as kuru and Creutzfeldt-Jakob disease. Studies also show that the brain attempts to repair its diseased circuits as old ones are ruined but that the natural repair structure is ultimately destroyed.

There is also a theory of aluminum intoxication which comes from findings that brains of people with Alzheimer's disease contain aluminum at levels up to thirty times those of normal, age-matched controls. Aluminum has already been implicated in the mental changes of dialysis dementia—a frequent side effect of long-term renal dialysis therapy. However, when scientists investigated such factors as the aluminum content of drinking water and use of aluminum pans by affected individuals, they concluded that there was no correlation. Moreover, aluminum workers do not have a higher rate of Alzheimer's disease than does the general population. Scientists do not know why aluminum builds up in patients with Alzheimer's disease, but they think it might actually represent an effect of the disease rather than a cause.

Some researchers feel that Alzheimer's disease may be due to the aging of the immune system. There have been findings of "anti-brain antibodies" in the blood of persons with the disease. It is thought that since the immune system occasionally goes haywire in the very old, the body may well be responding to its own cells, when they manifest age-related changes, as though they were foreign invaders. This could stimulate the formation of anti-brain antibodies, which are found in large numbers in the blood of the very old and in even larger numbers in patients with Alzheimer's disease.

Schizophrenia

Is there any possibility that there is a viral cause to schizophrenia?
Theories about a possible viral causation of schizophrenia have circulated in the medical community for more than a century, but research attempting to demonstrate a link has not been successful. However, Michael Harrington, a neurologist at the National Institute of Mental Health in Bethesda, Maryland, along with Carl R. Merril of NIMH and E. Fuller Torrey of St. Elizabeth's Hospital in Washington, D.C., have made a first step with their discovery of what appears to be a protein link in some schizophrenic patients. Through new techniques that detect trace amounts of protein, their research turned up two proteins in seventeen of fifty-four hospitalized schizophrenics that did not appear in any of ninety-nine healthy persons. The same two proteins, always appearing together, also have been found in a majority of patients with herpes simplex encephalitis and Creutzfeldt-Jakob disease, as well as in some patients with Parkinson's disease and multiple sclerosis. Although it is unknown what the presence of the proteins means, the data suggest that the proteins originate within the nervous systems of individuals whose illnesses involve the brain. A host of past studies into viral causes of schizophrenia have been inconclusive and often at odds with each other, but the connection between this disease and the appearance of the two proteins will certainly spark further research into the area.

chapter 7

When Immunity Fails and Bacteria Invade

Because we've known about bacterial diseases for longer than we have been aware of viral infections, and since bacteria are easier to combat than viruses, most people consider the more common bacterial diseases, if they ever even think about them at all, as contagious diseases that have been conquered. However, there are still many puzzles surrounding bacterial diseases. And, because many parents are neglecting to have their children immunized, cases of such diseases as diphtheria, whooping cough, and tuberculosis are again being seen. Understanding the history and nature of these diseases gives new insight into the great strides that have been made in treating immune system diseases in this century.

Diphtheria

What is diphtheria?
Known all over the world since the days of the ancient Hebrews but no longer common thanks to immunization, diphtheria is caused by diphtheria bacilli, which invade the tissues and liberate a poisonous substance called diphtheria toxin. The toxin destroys the cells lining the nose, throat, or larynx, producing a grayish membrane which congeals over the area. The uvula and tonsils swell, and the inflammation coats the area with a dirty grayish or yellowish-white membrane. Heart involvement is the most common complication of diphtheria, occurring in over 50 percent of diphtheria patients. Nerve paralysis, most commonly involving the soft palate and throat and sometimes the arms and legs, as

well as the eye and diaphragm muscles, sometimes occurs but usually lasts no more than 6 months.

In 1900 there were over 12,000 cases of diphtheria in the city of New York, resulting in death for the 25 percent who were not treated actively. Large-scale immunizations against diphtheria began between 1925 and 1927. Diphtheria is practically unheard of today, though small outbreaks and epidemics do occur, primarily in communities containing unimmunized or incompletely immunized persons.

Whooping Cough

What is whooping cough?
Whooping cough, also called pertussis, is a very contagious disease caused by bacteria known as *Bordetella pertussis*. It usually begins like a mild cold with a cough. After 10 or 14 days, the coughing begins to come in spells or bouts that are caused by an attempt to rid the system of thick mucus. Gagging and vomiting often occur following a bout of coughing. There are bursts of coughing in one breath, which force much of the air out of the lungs. Then, because of the lack of oxygen, a forcible noisy intake of air creates the crowing sound known as the whoop. This whooping stage usually lasts 3 or 4 weeks, after which attacks become less severe and less frequent, usually disappearing by the end of 6 weeks. Whooping cough is a serious disease, especially in children under 2 years of age. The main dangers are exhaustion and pneumonia.

What is a DPT shot?
A DPT shot is an inoculation against *d*iphtheria, *p*ertussis (whooping cough), and *t*etanus. The three materials are combined together and given in one shot. It is recommended that the inoculations be started early in life, preferably at 2 months of age. The series of shots (with each shot containing diphtheria, pertussis, and tetanus materials) are given three times, at intervals usually about 2 months apart. A booster shot is generally given a year later (at 15 to 18 months of age) to bring the protection back to a high level. Another booster is given again at 4 to 6 years of age. Further inoculations against diphtheria and tetanus are recommended every 10 years thereafter.

Does whooping cough vaccine produce reactions?
Whooping cough vaccine, made of killed whooping cough germs,

produces many more reactions than do diphtheria and tetanus toxoids. Sometimes an injection of whooping cough vaccine can cause a severe reaction, including high fever and, in rare instances, a convulsion. Because whooping cough is a dangerous disease for babies, inoculation is given early in life.

How soon is whooping cough vaccine effective?
Two or three shots must be administered before the vaccine stimulates the body to build immunity. No immediate help can be expected from a first inoculation given after a child has already been exposed to the disease. To maintain protection, booster shots are usually given at 15 months and 4 years.

Tetanus

What is tetanus?
Tetanus, or lockjaw, is a nervous system disease caused by the toxin of the bacillus *Clostridium tetani,* which is found in soil, dust, and the bowels of cows and horses. The tetanus bacterium is anaerobic, which means that it lives where oxygen is not present. It usually enters the body through wounds that are contaminated by soil or animal feces. The patient develops stiffness of the muscles and difficulty in opening his or her mouth (lockjaw). A wound is more likely to be infected with tetanus if it is deep. A deep puncture from a nail in a barnyard, for example, would be the riskiest kind. Many people think that the rust on a nail is the cause of tetanus. Actually, the tetanus germ occurs most frequently in soil and other places where horse and cow manure have been. Rust is not ordinarily a factor. If there is no proof that toxoid inoculations have been given and have had time to stimulate the buildup of antibodies, tetanus immune globulin (made from humans) or tetanus antitoxin serum (made from horses) will be given for temporary protection following a wound. This immunity is temporary. The horse-serum injection may produce serum sickness—hives and fever—a few weeks after it is given.

Tuberculosis

What is tuberculosis?
Tuberculosis (TB) is a widespread disease of humans—sometimes acute, often chronic—caused by tubercle bacilli. The bacteria usually enter the body through the air passages, though they may

be ingested when food or drink is infected. The curved rod of the tubercle bacillus is found in both humans and bovine animals, and the pasteurization of milk and the use of tuberculin-tested cows helped to reduce the spread of the disease. When judiciously used, antituberculosis antibiotics and chemicals—including ethambutol, isoniazid, streptomycin, and rifampin—can now achieve recovery in nearly every case of pulmonary tuberculosis.

The bacteria usually invade lung tissues or the lymph nodes draining the lung area, and can enter the blood to be carried to organs in any part of the body. Sometimes bacteria are walled off by the body's immune defense and remain dormant for months, years, or a lifetime.

When tuberculosis infection occurs, it is often unrecognized, frequently being mistaken for the flu or other minor illness. There may be fever and cough, and perhaps a little pain in the chest. The signs of primary infection that has healed are found in a large proportion of healthy people. If secondary tuberculous infection occurs, or tubercle bacilli spread from the primary focus, the symptoms may include spitting of blood, a chronic cough, pain in the chest on breathing, tiredness, loss of appetite, night sweats, and cessation of menstrual periods in women. As the disease progresses, the patient loses weight. Lymph glands may be enlarged. The disease may spread to the bones, causing pain in diseased joints—often the knees, hips, or spine. Tuberculosis in the kidneys, bladder, testicles, or prostate gland causes symptoms similar to those of urogenital infections.

What is the vaccine used for tuberculosis?

BCG is the name of the tuberculosis vaccine. The initials stand for "the bacillus of Calmette and Guerin," two French scientists. The vaccine is made from tubercle bacilli that have been weakened by being transferred from one culture medium to another repeatedly over a long time. The tubercle bacilli retain most of their usual characteristics, except the ability to produce generalized tuberculosis. When injected, instead of spreading through the body, the vaccine produces a small nodule in the arm or leg where it is injected. This infection is mild and remains localized, yet it produces an immunity to the germ.

What is the purpose of the skin test for tuberculosis?

A "tine test" for tuberculosis has been used for routine testing. The tines are several tiny sharp plastic points that protrude from a plastic base. The tines, coated with tuberculin, are pressed briefly into the skin. This method is less painful than injecting tuberculin with a hypodermic needle. If no red spot develops, the body has not been infected with tuberculosis germs. Anyone who has ever had a tuberculosis infection will react with a positive test result for the rest of his or her life, even though the infection has healed.

How has the incidence of tuberculosis been affected by the use of antituberculosis antibiotics and vaccine?

In the early 1900s, over 80 percent of the population was infected with tuberculosis *before* the age of 20. A 1946 autopsy study showed evidence of tuberculosis in 80 percent of persons over the age of 50. In 1978, only 2 to 5 percent of young adults reacted to tuberculin (except in some urban areas), and 25 percent of persons over the age of 50 reacted. The great improvement is due to the fact that fewer people have infectious cases of tuberculosis, the standard of living has improved, there is a reduced risk of late progression of infection, and recognition and treatment of infectious cases is prompt and effective. The dramatic change in the status of tuberculosis can be appreciated by a comparison of mortality rates. Once the leading cause of death, responsible for 200 deaths per 100,000 in 1906, in 1976 tuberculosis was listed as the cause of death in only 1.5 deaths per 100,000.

Old Remedies for Tuberculosis

Roman authors suggested wolf's liver boiled in wine, elephant's blood, or—if necessary—a bath in the urine of a person who had eaten cabbage.

In the fourteenth century, weasel blood and pigeon droppings were the usual prescriptions for tuberculosis. All else failing, it was advised that the patient "betake himself to the king," because the mere touch of royalty was believed to heal tuberculosis of the lymph nodes in the neck.

English monarchs—from Edward the Confessor to Queen Anne, who died in 1714—were available for "touching" to cure disease. Samuel Johnson, when he was aged 2, was touched by Queen Anne for tuberculosis of the lymph nodes in the neck and proudly wore the touchpiece for the rest of his life. Actually, tuberculous lymph nodes of childhood usually heal spontaneously, so monarchs' reputations were safeguarded by nature.

Typhoid Fever

What is typhoid fever?
Typhoid fever is caused by a short, plump, rod-shaped bacterium called *Salmonella typhosa,* which produces infection in humans only when it enters the alimentary tract. After a patient has had the disease—even in a very mild form—the bacteria may survive in the gallbladder for years, so that the patient becomes a carrier. Symptoms of the disease start after an incubation period of 1 to 2 weeks. The patient has headaches, feels ill and dizzy, has pains in the limbs and sometimes a sore throat and cough. Bleeding of the nose and a slow pulse are usually present. The tongue becomes sore and cheeks are flushed. A rash may develop, consisting of rose spots on the abdomen and thorax. Bleeding from ulcers in the wall of the small intestine sometimes occurs. At this point, the patient may go into a typhoid state, with low muttering delirium. Stools become loose, and many typhoid bacilli are released in stool and urine, making the patient highly infectious. Death occurs in 10 to 15 percent of patients. Immunization by injection of a combined vaccine containing heat-killed *Salmonella typhi* and *S. paratyphi* A and B (T.A.B. vaccine) has helped to reduce the mortality from typhoid from a high of between 72 and 134 per 100,000 in the 1860s to 31.3 per 100,000 in 1900 and to zero in the 1970s.

Who was Typhoid Mary?
At least fifty-nine cases of typhoid fever and three deaths were traced to the now-famous Irish cook, Mary Mallon, better known as Typhoid Mary. She was picked up by a vigilant health department officer, George Soper, in 1906 when he traced six cases of typhoid to a household where she had been a cook for 3 weeks. By the time she was located she had caused seven epidemics in the space of 6 years. When she would not allow herself to be examined, the Health Department placed her in a hospital, where numerous examinations showed that she was a living culture tube. She was released after promising not to seek employment that involved handling food, and she disappeared for 5 years. When she was again discovered, at the end of another trail of epidemics, she was placed in a hospital where she remained until she died 23 years later. (When she sued for release, the courts and much of the press supported the Health Department's action.) Other carriers of the disease were persuaded to have their gallbladders

removed, since doctors had found that typhoid bacilli lodged in the gallbladder of chronic carriers and that when the gallbladder was removed, the stools often remained permanently free of the bacilli.

Scarlet Fever

What is scarlet fever?
Scarlet fever, also known as scarlatina, is characterized by a sore throat and pinprick red skin rash that causes superficial flaking after it disappears. It is primarily due to group A hemolytic streptococci. The disease is much less common now than in the past because of the use of penicillin, though immune-complex nephritis and rheumatic fever are complications that may occur.

Although scarlet fever was clearly defined as a disease in 1861, its cause was in dispute until 1924 because the streptococci that were found in throats of scarlet fever victims could also be cultured from the throats of healthy persons. The streptococci could not be cultivated from the skin that peeled after the rash, nor could they be found in the blood. Scarlet fever is produced by one type of streptococcus—the same infection that produces tonsillitis, sore throats, swollen glands, and some ear infections. If a person develops a sore throat caused by a strain of group A hemolytic streptococci that produces erythrogenic toxin and the person has no immunity to the toxin, he or she will have scarlet fever. If the person is immune to the toxin or if the particular strain of streptococci does not produce the toxin, he or she will have a sore throat without a rash, or streptococcal sore throat. If the streptococcus to which the person is immune lodges in the throat, he or she will most likely not develop any illness. This explains why in a single epidemic, some persons will have scarlet fever and others only streptococcal sore throat. The Dick test for scarlet fever injects a small amount of erythrogenic toxin. Reddening of the skin within 24 to 48 hours indicates susceptibility to scarlet fever.

Rheumatic Fever

What is rheumatic fever?
A disease that affects the joints, heart, and nervous system, rheumatic fever is caused by an abnormal response to group A hemolytic streptococci. Joint pains, followed by heart and pericardial

disease, and the presence of Aschoff's nodules in various tissues, are accepted as positive evidence of rheumatic fever. It is believed that products of hemolytic streptococci produce an allergic reaction in certain tissues, thereby causing malfunction and, in the case of the heart, lasting damage. Rheumatic fever is an extremely variable disease, sometimes taking an acute form with high fever, sometimes smoldering for weeks with little or no fever symptoms. It can recur again and again whenever there is another streptococcal infection. There are several drugs effective in clearing up streptococcal infections and in hastening the end of rheumatic inflammation in joints and heart.

Is there a streptococcus vaccine?
Not yet. There are about eighty strains of the streptococcus bacteria that cause painful sore throats. Genetically produced proteins differ from strain to strain, making it difficult to devise a vaccine that will cover a variety of streptococcus bacteria. However, understanding of the workings of streptococcus may make development of a vaccine possible in the future.

Meningitis and Pneumonia

Is meningitis caused by bacteria?
Meningitis, the inflammation of the three membranes enveloping the brain and spinal cord, can be caused by the invasion of the central nervous system by one of a number of organisms—including bacteria and viruses. It often follows diseases of viral origin such as mumps and diseases caused by Coxsackie viruses.

What is pneumonia?
Pneumonia is an inflammation of the lungs that usually starts with a virus or bacterium, but may be caused by fungi, such as molds, and chemical irritants. Difficult breathing, along with a dry cough and fever, are early symptoms.

Bacterial pneumonia is caused by bacteria such as *streptococcus pneumoniae* and *staphylococcus aureus*. Antibiotics are given as soon as the diagnosis of bacterial pneumonia is made, and though it is in some cases a serious disease, the majority of patients respond quickly to treatment. Viral pneumonia is caused by a number of viruses that may infect the air passages and the lungs, such as adenoviruses, or influenza, parainfluenza, smallpox, and varicella viruses. Although it can produce a fatal infection, usually this type of pneumonia is less severe than bacterial pneumonia. A new strain of the disease, discovered in 1976 and known as Legionnaires' disease because most of the victims were attending an American Legion convention at a large hotel, was finally identified as being caused by a bacteria that bred in the unsanitary water in shower drains and air conditioners.

Are there vaccines available for pneumonia and meningitis?
Recent research has focused on developing vaccines that use only part of an infectious agent. Called subunit vaccines, these are now available for pneumonia and meningitis. They produce the desired immunity without stirring up separate immune reactions to the many antigens carried, for instance, on a single bacterium.

What is HIB vaccine?
This is a new vaccine which gives lifelong immunity to some pneumonia strains. It is being added to routine vaccinations given to children between the ages of 2 and 5.

Gonorrhea

What is gonorrhea?
Gonorrhea is a bacterial disease that affects the sexual organs. Both men and women are susceptible to gonorrhea, although 85 percent of infected women have no apparent symptoms. In women, gonorrhea can spread into the cervix and pelvic cavity, scarring the fallopian tubes and impairing fertility. If a pregnant woman has gonorrhea, the child's eyes may be infected during delivery. Untreated, the infection can cause blindness in the child.

The major symptom of gonorrhea in men is a discharge of pus from the penis, accompanied by a burning sensation during urination. Any person who suspects infection should seek treatment immediately and should warn all sexual partners of the possibility of infection. Gonorrhea can be cured by treatment with penicillin and other antibiotics.

Has a vaccine been developed for gonorrhea?
Scientists have been trying to develop a vaccine against the bacteria called gonococci for a quarter of a century, and an experimental vaccine is presently being tested to assess its safety and ability to produce immunity. However, many ex-

perts believe it will be many more years before an effective vaccine is developed, proved, and introduced for use. The strain of bacteria that causes gonorrhea is particularly adept at evolving ways of eluding the antibodies the body produces to fight it. The bacteria produce an enzyme that can slice antibodies apart, destroying their effectiveness. Even though the complete process is unknown, scientists have puzzled out some of the details of how the bacteria circumvent the body's immune defenses and infect human cells. Vaccine researchers are using these discoveries in developing new strategies to try to crack the gonorrhea puzzle. Using advanced techniques of molecular biology, Dr. Gary Schoolnick of Stanford University and his colleagues have prepared synthetic chains of amino acids, known as peptides, linking them to natural protein from the outer membrane of the bacteria. It is hoped that in the near future a combination vaccine will be available for gonorrhea and meningitis. Chemically and biologically, meningitis and gonorrhea have much in common.

Syphilis

What is syphilis?
Syphilis is an infectious, chronic venereal disease caused by a spirochete (a spiral-shaped bacterium). It can be transmitted by direct contact or congenitally. It usually progresses in three stages of increasing severity: primary, with a hard sore on the infected part; secondary, involving a secondary rash and blood changes; and tertiary, which involves every system of the body, including the brain.

chapter 8

Other Immunity Failures

Besides the viral and bacterial diseases that are well understood, there are other disease villains of several types that also come under the immune-disease umbrella. These include autoimmune diseases, in which the immune system attacks the body, and immune deficiency diseases, in which a component of the immune system is missing or has become deficient, resulting in serious health problems. In some cases, the cause of a disease is unknown and research efforts to discover bacterial, viral, or fungal agents are ongoing. Facing the future, it is comforting to know that we are armed with the sophisticated tools of new research in genetic technology.

Why is it that new diseases are always being discovered?
The question is whether we are noticing new diseases because we have modern techniques with which to detect and evaluate them— or whether technology and its effects on our lifestyles play a role in encouraging the development of new diseases. In the past decade, Legionnaires' disease, Lyme arthritis, and toxic shock syndrome have been in the headlines. Trips to remote parts of the world bring travelers into contact with many diseases that have either been eliminated from our society or were never present or common within it. Throughout history there have been many diseases of epidemic proportion that appeared suddenly, ravaged a population, and eventually disappeared, leaving scientists baffled. New technologies, coupled with great advances in modern medical understanding, make it possible for scientists to more quickly identify, classify, and attempt to treat new diseases.

Allergies

What is an allergy?
An allergy is a sensitivity to a substance that in similar amounts is harmless to other people.

What is an allergen?
An allergen is an antigen that causes an overreaction or sensitive reaction within the body. It may be animal, mineral, or vegetable. The list of known allergens includes everything from cat hairs to the sun, from milk to eggshells.

What causes allergic reactions?
Allergic reactions are false alarms being answered by the immune system. A normally harmless substance is perceived as a threat and attacked. The immune system cannot distinguish between dangerous intruders such as bacteria or parasites and innocent ones such as grass pollen or house dust, or even beneficial ones such as milk or eggs. If the material is perceived as foreign, the immune system goes on to attack.

How are allergies related to the immune system?
The wheezing, sneezing, runny nose, itchy eyes, rashes, and bumps that characterize allergic reactions are the result of the immune system responding to a false alarm. In a susceptible person, a normally harmless substance—such as pollen, cat hair, or dust—is perceived as a threat and then attacked by the immune system. When allergic people are first exposed to an antigen or allergen, their bodies produce large amounts of the corresponding antibody. These IgE immunoglobulin molecules attach to the surfaces of mast cells in tissue or basophils in the circulation. When an IgE antibody positioned on a mast cell or basophil encounters its specific allergen, the IgE antibody signals the mast cell or basophil to release the powerful chemicals inside it. It is these chemical mediators that cause the allergic symptoms.

What happens to the body when a person has an allergy?
The allergic person develops an antibody aimed at a specific irritant (the allergen). When this antibody comes in contact with the allergen, the body attacks, histamine is released, and inflammation begins. If histamine is released in the nostrils, eyelids, or lining of the bronchial tubes, the swelling and itching cause sneezing, a runny nose, stuffiness, itchy eyes, or coughing and wheezing.

Are there any new treatments for controlling allergies?
There are several treatments that are only available under a doctor's supervision. They include the following:

- A new type of antihistamine, terfenadine, is less likely to cause drowsiness than other antihistamines.
- A drug, cromolyn sodium, available as nasal spray or eyedrops, inhibits the release of histamine from cells in the nasal passages and eyes. Different from antihistamines, which block histamine's subsequent effects, this drug, if used before exposure to allergens, can often prevent symptoms.
- Steroid derivatives beclomethasone dipropionate and flunisolide, available as nasal sprays, counteract nasal swelling and congestion.
- New immunotherapy, or a series of allergy shots, can be given in larger doses than were previously available, over a shorter period of time. The shots build tolerance to specific allergens and are effective against pollen and dust allergies but not against mold allergies.

Scientists at the National Institute of Allergic and Infectious Diseases are working on some long-range possibilities against allergies. One is a way to turn off production of IgE, the antibody implicated in most allergies. The other is a way of killing off or stabilizing mast cells, cells that are found where the body is open to foreign agents: in the linings of the nose and throat, the intestine, the skin, or the blood. This approach tries to keep the mast cells from releasing histamine and other mediators that cause an allergic reaction.

What is hay fever?
Hay fever does not come from hay, nor does it cause a fever. Its technical name is *allergic rhinitis,* meaning an allergic inflammation of the nose. Any of a combination of several allergens may cause hay fever. Known allergens include timothy, orchard grasses, oak pollen, spring sycamore, birch, hickory, beech, maple, elder, and cedar pollens, as well as ragweed pollen, tumbleweed, marsh elder, hemp, cocklebur, and thistle. Those who have hay fever on a year-round basis may find that their hay fever is caused by some foods, dusts, animal danders, molds, perfumes, hairsprays, or other household

products. When hay fever symptoms are caused by this last group of allergens, the condition is described by physicians as perennial allergic rhinitis.

Hay fever is the most common allergy in the United States. Its symptoms include itchy eyes, runny nose, itchy red skin, headaches, congestion, fatigue, swelling, coughing, sneezing, and wheezing. For some, hay fever is just a nuisance. For others, it's a disabling chronic illness.

What is asthma and who gets it?

Three out of every hundred people in the Western world suffer from asthma, America's second most common allergic disease. In other parts of the world—in West Africa or among New Zealand highlanders and Eskimos, for example—it is rarely reported. Asthma is characterized by repeated sudden attacks of shortness of breath and audible wheezing. Most attacks are short, lasting minutes to hours, and after them the patient seems to recover completely. Some cases of asthma are caused by bronchial allergies to airborne substances; however, aspirin, environmental factors, occupational factors, infections, vigorous exercise, and emotional stress are also known to provoke attacks. In any event, the result of the attack is a response by the immune system, which causes the symptoms of asthma.

Does asthma last a lifetime?

Not always. About one-third of the people with asthma are children, and about half of them will outgrow the illness, for unknown reasons. In general, asthma attacks are less severe, less frequent, and less permanent in people who develop the illness at an early age. The exception is asthma in children under 2. Since it has so many causes, no single drug works well against asthma in every case. The disease is treated with a variety of drugs, often in combination. In cases of asthma triggered by allergic reactions, the best approach is to pinpoint the cause of the allergy and avoid it if possible.

What is pneumonitis?

The condition known as pneumonitis, allergic alveolitis, allergic pneumonia, or hypersensitivity pneumonitis—all referring to the same disease—is characterized by an inflammation of the lungs, reflecting an immunologic reaction at several locations within the lungs. There is an acute and a chronic form of pneumonitis. The acute form of the disease is characterized by chills, fever, malaise, labored breathing, and cough within 2 to 8 hours after exposure to an allergen—such as hay, mushrooms, malt, or fur, to name just a few possibilities. In the chronic form of the disease the patient is fatigued and has labored breathing and a nonproductive cough over a period of time.

How do foods cause allergic reactions?

Immune mechanisms are involved, the result of sensitization of IgE antibodies, similar to the sensitization process in hayfever. Cow's milk, egg whites, wheat, corn, seafood, chocolate, and nuts are common foods which produce allergic reactions. Legumes, including peanuts, peas, beans, soybeans, and licorice (which is classified as a leguminous herb) are also associated with allergic reactions. Hundreds of foods and food additives are known to stimulate allergic reactions in humans.

Dr. May believes that proper controls should be used in allergy testing of foods so that clinical observations are not distorted by psychological influences. He notes that in recent scientific studies of persons giving impressive histories of reactions to foods, only about one-third of the histories could be confirmed in double-blind challenges—that is, when neither the patient nor the observer knew what food was being consumed.

What is anaphylactic shock?

Anaphylactic shock results when the immune system completely overreacts to a foreign substance, causing death in a matter of minutes. It is most commonly seen in cases of bee stings or in those who react violently to antibiotics such as penicillin. Very few deaths actually occur each year from these causes, but each case is evidence of the power, potency, and possible lethal effects of an immune system misreading its foe.

Autoimmune Diseases

What are autoimmune diseases?

The term *autoimmune* describes a group of diseases in which the immune system attacks the body. An abnormal production of antibodies is thought to be at fault. Rheumatoid arthritis is believed to involve this abnormal autoimmune action. Antibodies against the patient's own tissues can be found in the joints swollen by rheumatoid arthritis. Systemic lupus erythematosus also seems to involve antibodies directed against the patient's own tissues.

Arthritis

Is arthritis really a disease of the immune system?
Since inflammation is the body's defense reaction to any form of injury, diseases that involve inflammatory processes in the body have a relationship to the immune system. Sometimes the immune system fails to distinguish self from nonself and thus attacks its own tissues. This self-destruction plays a role in arthritis. Arthritis appears in more than 100 forms, including rheumatoid arthritis, one of the two most common varieties and the most destructive and crippling form, gout, and systemic lupus erythematosus (SLE), which is also considered a form of arthritis. Osteoarthritis, the other most common type, researchers believe, is not a disease of the immune system. Rather, it is a "wear and tear" disease, considered mechanical rather than systemic.

What is rheumatoid arthritis?
Most researchers believe that rheumatoid arthritis is largely a disorder of the immune system in which the system attacks the body's own cells as if they were invading microorganisms. Some think it is caused by a virus infection, a one-celled organism, or a dietary deficiency. It is a mysterious disease about which scientists are learning more every day.

Rheumatoid arthritis has two levels. One is inflammation of joints and tissue around the joints. The other, which is more serious, is destruction of joints, tendons, ligaments, and cartilage. Most of the medicine now available relieves the pain and swelling of the disease but cannot control its destructive aspects. Many people never suffer the crippling aspects of arthritis. Only a small percentage are afflicted with the most serious form.

What research is being done on rheumatoid arthritis?
Researchers from the University of California at San Francisco, along with colleagues at Massachusetts General Hospital in Boston, reported that they were able to increase the severity of experimentally induced arthritis in rats by injecting a neurotransmitter—a substance that transmits nerve impulses in the brain—into joints. This was the first direct evidence that the ner-

vous system is involved in rheumatoid arthritis and that a nervous system substance contributes to the symptoms and joint destruction of arthritis.

Other scientists are investigating whether sensitivity to certain foods causes the joints to react. While treating overweight patients, doctors at Wayne State University in Detroit found that a low-fat diet helped some who had rheumatoid arthritis. Other studies have discovered that specific foods prompt flare-ups. Researchers at the University of Washington in Seattle treated patients with zinc, which helped reduce joint pain, swelling, and stiffness. (In Israel, two doctors found that vitamin E provided some relief to people with osteoarthritis.) For many, aspirin still remains the preferred treatment, since it can reduce the inflammation of rheumatoid arthritis and kill pain. For those who cannot use aspirin, a variety of aspirinlike drugs, called nonsteroidal anti-inflammatory drugs, are used. Exercise has also proven useful for arthritis.

Are any new treatments being offered to people with rheumatoid arthritis?
Two treatments that have come out of the cancer field are being tested for rheumatoid arthritis. Gamma interferon has shown results in studies conducted in West Germany and the United States. One of a class of rare, naturally occurring proteins that biotechnology concerns have produced using genetic engineering techniques, gamma interferon, in preliminary trials, lessened the pain, swollen joints, and other problems of arthritis patients.

Methotrexate, researchers at the Harvard Medical School have discovered, can provide relief to some patients. Long used to treat patients with breast, lung, head, and neck cancers, methotrexate relieved some pain and swelling for more than half the patients studied.

A third treatment, a drug called interleukin-1 blocker, is in the early stages of development.

Has arthritis been known throughout history?
Arthritis is known to have made life miserable for Alexander the Great and for Julius Caesar. It forced Henry VI to postpone his wedding day. The immortal artist Benvenuto Cellini suffered from arthritis, as did many members of the Medici family. Skeletons of Neanderthal men showed that spines were deformed by osteoarthritis. Egyptian writings dating back 6000 years contain de-

scriptions of treatments for rheumatoid arthritis. Even the skeletons of dinosaurs, dating back 200 million years, show evidence of osteoarthritis.

Lupus

What is lupus?

Lupus, which is Latin for *wolf*, has been described in medical literature since the time of Hippocrates, when the disease was characterized as causing a skin condition that made it look as though the patient had been bitten by a ravenous wolf. This type of lupus, sometimes called lupus vulgaris, is known more accurately today as cutaneous tuberculosis. Thanks to medication dealing with the tuberculosis bacillus, lupus vulgaris no longer causes the devastation it once did.

The immune system disease known as lupus (scientifically referred to as lupus erythematosus) is a disease that involves the entire immune system and connective tissue. It can affect the skin (discoid lupus erythematosus) or it can strike the blood, joints, central nervous system, or kidneys (systemic lupus erythematosus). Encompassing the entire spectrum of the body's responses to antigens, systemic lupus causes chronic inflammation and the attack of the body's defense mechanisms against its own cells. Lupus exists in many forms, ranging from very mild to severe. In its extreme form, lupus actively mobilizes the body against itself.

How does systemic lupus differ from many other immune system diseases?

While it displays many of the characteristics of inflammatory processes found in infections, lupus persists—or may come and go unpredictably—as a chronic condition. While antibodies are active in lupus, their activity seems to be completely misdirected—causing the destruction of the body's own tissues. About 90 percent of lupus sufferers are women, most in the childbearing years from the teens to the forties.

Are there any known causes of lupus?

In 10 to 12 percent of diagnosed lupus cases, it appears that the patient may be allergic to a drug. A number of different types of medication have been found to set off the lupus process. These include procainamide (Procan, Pronestyl), a drug used to correct cardiac irregularities; hydralazine (Apresoline), a drug used to treat high blood pressure; sulfonamides, the so-called sulfa drugs, used to treat infections; nitrofurantoin, used for urinary tract infections; and tetracycline and other biosynthetic antibiotics, which cause problems when outdated or improperly stored under conditions of high heat and humidity. Some tranquilizers and anti convulsants and penicillamine, a drug used to treat rheumatoid arthritis, have also been implicated. However, in most cases, the cause of the cellular destruction is unknown.

What are the symptoms of lupus?
Persistent aching of the joints—fingers, knuckles, wrists, or knees; rashes, often on the face, shoulders, and arms, sometimes forming a butterfly pattern over the bridge of the nose and cheeks; fatigue; heart problems; anemia; weight loss; kidney and sensory malfunction; false-positive tests for syphilis; sun sensitivity; pleurisy; pneumonia; hair loss; mental and emotional problems; nausea and vomiting; and jaundice have all been listed as symptoms of lupus. Most people first visit a doctor because of puzzling symptoms involving the skin or mucous membranes, aches in joints, low or persistent fever, and sun sensitivity. Hair loss, cardiac problems, pleuritis or pleurisy, and major kidney-function abnormalities usually occur during the course of the illness.

What happens to DNA in lupus patients?
Antibodies to DNA (known as anti-dsDNA) are found frequently in active stages of lupus and in 70 to 80 percent of all lupus patients at some time, but only occasionally in other conditions. Antibodies to single-stranded DNA can be found in about 90 percent of lupus patients, but are also found in patients with rheumatoid arthritis and other connective-tissue disorders. Some studies have indicated that anti-dsDNA is not usually found in patients who do not have lupus. Immunologists are experimenting with monoclonal antibodies to arrest a disease in mice that resembles lupus and are finding that helper T cells are important in the development of mouse autoimmune disease.

Colitis

What is colitis?
Colitis is a chronic inflammation and ulceration of the colon and rectum. There are two types of chronic inflammatory bowel disease: chronic nonspecific ulcerative colitis and granulomatous

colitis, known as Crohn's disease. The two share many clinical, pathologic, and epidemiologic features. Both diseases are more common in whites than in nonwhites, in urban than in rural settings, in Jews than in non-Jews. In cases of nonspecific ulcerative colitis, the patient, usually a young adult, develops diarrhea and bleeding, which may give way to constipation. In time, diarrhea becomes the principal symptom. There is abdominal pain and tenderness, and when the condition is severe, dehydration may occur.

What is Crohn's disease?

Crohn's disease, also known as regional enteritis, is a chronic inflammatory disorder that may involve any portion of the gastrointestinal tract—the esophagus, stomach, duodenum, jejunum, and ileum. A similar inflammatory condition may occur in the colon, either alone or with accompanying small-intestinal colitis, and is referred to as Crohn's disease of the colon. Though the cause is unknown, the search continues for an infectious basis for the disease. In spite of numerous attempts to find known bacterial, fungal, or viral agents, none has thus far been isolated. Research has been carried out to determine whether the disease can be transferred to laboratory animals by injecting extracts of the diseased tissues into the animals. A granulomatous inflammatory reaction, similar to Crohn's disease, has been produced in the footpads of mice following injections. The theory that an immune mechanism may be involved is based on the concept that other manifestations of the disease—arthritis and pericholangitis—may represent autoimmune responses and that corticosteroids and azathioprine, which are successfully used in treating the disease, may exert their effects through immunosuppressive mechanisms. In a small group of patients, the original complaint is acute pain in the right lower quadrant, suggestive of acute appendicitis.

What indications are there that ulcerative colitis and Crohn's disease are caused by an immune system problem?

The serum of some patients with ulcerative colitis contains an antibody to colon epithelial cells. It is thought that this antibody probably results from tissue injury, and it has also been found in patients with a number of unrelated gastrointestinal diseases. Peripheral lymphocytes from patients with both chronic ulcerative colitis and Crohn's disease of the colon are cytotoxic to colon epithelial cells grown in tissue culture. Lymphocytes from patients with either disorder also release a substance that inhibits macrophage migration.

Immune Deficiency Diseases

How are immune deficiency diseases caused?

Lack of one or more components of the immune system results in an immune deficiency disease. Deficiencies can be inherited, acquired through illness, or produced as an inadvertent side effect of certain drug treatments. People with advanced cancer may have immune deficiencies as a result of either the disease or the treatments. Immune deficiencies can develop in the wake of common viral infections such as influenza, mononucleosis, and measles. Blood transfusions, malnutrition, and stress can also cause immune deficiencies.

Does the problem of Rh-factor incompatibility relate to the immunologic system?

Yes. *Erythroblastosis fetalis* is the medical term for the anemia that results in the Rh-positive fetus or newborn infant of an Rh-negative mother. Rh is a blood type. The problem arises when a woman who has Rh-negative blood conceives a child with a man who has Rh-positive blood. Generally the first baby born to an Rh-negative mother has no problems. However, if that baby's father has Rh-positive blood and if the baby's blood is Rh positive, a few of the baby's red blood cells escape into the mother's circulation and sensitize her immune system against blood of that type. In the course of the next pregnancy with a fetus of the Rh-positive blood type, the mother's internal defense system destroys Rh-positive blood cells, resulting in fatal anemia in the fetus. The Rh factor wasn't discovered until 1940, and it wasn't until the 1960s that immunologists discovered that the key to the disease was the sensitizing of the mother against Rh-positive blood.

Are sprue and celiac disease immune system diseases?

Though research findings at this time are insufficient to definitely determine a relationship to the immune system, there are indications of possible immune system involvement in both diseases. People with nontropical sprue have an intolerance to a protein found in wheat and wheat products. Celiac disease in children produces the same symptoms. HLA-B8 antigen has been found in 85 to 90 percent of sprue patients, as compared with 20 to 25 percent of normal patients. It is believed that the HLA-B8 antigen is linked to immune-response genes that may determine the immunologic recognition of certain substances. Such genetic factors may predispose a person to immunologic intolerance of dietary proteins such as the peptides in gluten or to the production of pathogenic antigluten antibodies that could result in binding of gluten to the lining of the intestine, with subsequent tissue damage. It has been found that when gluten is introduced into the ilea of sprue patients, changes begin to occur within hours. These changes are confined to the ileum and do not affect the upper jejunum, suggesting that the effect is immediate and local rather than systemic. Further research is needed to determine the exact cause of gluten intolerance.

Can zinc help patients with sprue and celiac disease?

There have been some studies of patients with sprue or celiac disease who failed to respond to diet, steroids, or nutritional supplements but did gain weight and have improved absorption when given zinc. Some patients who had absorption problems other than those associated with celiac disease also had beneficial results from supplementation of zinc.

What is toxic shock syndrome?

Toxic shock syndrome is caused by a toxin (TSST-1) produced by a common bacterium known as *staphylococcus aureus*—which also causes cystitis, osteomyelitis, endocarditis, and pneumonia, as well as pimples and food poisoning. It has been discovered that when levels of magnesium are relatively high, the bacteria produces little of the toxin. When levels of magnesium are low, toxin levels rise, causing the bacteria to produce toxin. Researchers at Harvard Medical School report that polyester foam and polyacrylate rayon, the two substances that are known to foster the production of TSST-1, are no longer being used in the manufacture of tampons, though some surgical dressings contain the two fibers. Toxic shock syndrome, originally believed to occur only in menstruating women, has been seen under a wide variety of circumstances—including in women following surgery or birth, people with abrasions, and those who use contraceptive sponges or diaphragms.

Symptoms of toxic shock syndrome include fever over 102°, low blood pressure or dizziness, and a skin rash. If recognized early, toxic shock syndrome can be treated with appropriate antibiotics. Delayed diagnosis can prove fatal. All but 5 percent of the population produce antibodies to toxic shock toxin. Only those who lack the antibodies are susceptible to the syndrome.

Index

About the Authors

Eve Potts, a medical writer, and Marion Morra, Assistant Director of the Yale University Comprehensive Cancer Center, are authors of *CHOICES: Realistic Alternatives in Cancer Treatment*, the best-selling book for cancer patients, their families and friends. Known for their ability to translate technical medical material into easy-to-understand language, the widely published authors are also editors of *The Cancer Prevention Letter*, a monthly publication, and of numerous National Cancer Institute and American Cancer Society patient education booklets. The sisters live and work in Connecticut.

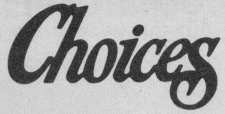

"Useful, illuminating, even life-saving information."
Los Angeles Times

WOMANCARE:
A GYNECOLOGICAL GUIDE TO YOUR BODY
**Lynda Madaras and
Jane Patterson, M.D., F.A.C.O.G.
with Peter Schick, M.D., F.A.C.S.**

Written with a deep and compassionate understanding of
women's special physical and emotional needs, this
encyclopedic work goes further than any other book to give
you a full range of information, treatments and alternatives—
to allow you to choose the one with which you are most
comfortable, and enable you to share more fully with your
doctor the responsibility and care of your own health. It
contains the most up-to-date material on the break-throughs
in technique and research that are revolutionizing women's
health care and treatment almost daily.

960 pages and over 100 charts and drawings give you detailed
information on self-examination, menstruation and meno-
pause, birth controls—safety, effectiveness and long-term
effects of all options—doctor-patient relationships, DES and
fertility drugs, and much, much more. A 500-page section on
diseases covers everything from minor infections to cancer.

"invaluable...Well organized, complete and easy to
understand...The most comprehensive gynecology text
published to date." *Library Journal*

"Impressive... WOMANCARE is a full-scale reference work.
...Women thus informed will know and like themselves better,
recognize bad medical care and have the ammunition to
stand up to their doctors when necessary. *Savvy*

AVON Trade Paperback   87643-4/$9.95

Available wherever paperbacks are sold or directly from the
publisher. Include $1.00 per copy for postage and handling; allow
6-8 weeks for delivery. Avon Books, Dept. BP, Box 767, Rte 2,
Dresden, TN 38225.

Womancare 4-85

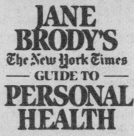